THE RAW FOOD GOURMET

THE RAW FOOD GOURMET

GOING RAW FOR TOTAL WELL-BEING

GABRIELLE CHAVEZ

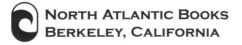

NORTH ATLANTIC BOOKS
BERKELEY, CALIFORNIA

Published by
North Atlantic Books
P.O. Box 12327
Berkeley, California 94712, USA

Published in the UK and Europe by Findhorn Press, 2005

Cover design by Paula Morrison
Text design by Thierry Bogliolo
Edited by Kate Keogan
Printed in the Unites States of America
Distributed to the book trade by Publishers Group West

The Raw Food Gourmet: Going Raw for Total Well-Being is sponsored by the Society for the Study of Native Arts and Sciences, a nonprofit educational corporation whose goals are to develop an educational and crosscultural perspective linking various scientific, social, and artistic fields; to nurture a holistic view of arts, sciences, humanities, and healing; and to publish and distribute literature on the relationship of mind, body, and nature.

Library of Congress Cataloging-in-Publication Data
Chavez, Gabrielle Fackre, 1953–
    The raw food gourmet : going raw for total well-being / by Gabrielle Fackre Chavez.
        p. cm.
        Includes bibliographical references and index.
        ISBN 1-55643-613-0 (pbk.)
    1. Cookery (Natural foods) 2. Raw foods. I. Title.
        TX741.C464 2005
        641.5'636--dc22
                                                                2005012910

1 2 3 4 5 6 7 8 9 UNITED 10 09 08 07 06 05

CONTENTS

TO SEEKERS EVERYWHERE

Acknowledgments

Some say that writing a book is like having a child. I agree that it is a labor, but there were a lot more people involved in the conception and delivery of this book than that other most personal of human activities. I do thank my husband Thomas who encouraged and supported me in every possible way to bring this to birth. Ben and Gilowen, my sons, have not only been willing to taste recipes, but have also inspired my forthcoming raw children's book, *Some People Think My Mom is Weird.*

Without the inspiration, information and wonderful food provided for us by the "Raw Family," Victoria, Igor, Sergei and Valya Boutenko, it is unlikely I would have made the transition to a 100% raw energy life at all. Heartfelt gratitude to you and to everyone in the blossoming raw foods community.

Everything I do is in community, and I wish to recognize the members of my spiritual community, Christ the Healer United Church of Christ in Portland, Oregon, for the diversity of gifts they shared with me, beginning with the enthusiasm for raw foods that several members first brought to us. I appreciate the gift of willingness to embrace my enthusiasm in turn that the community demonstrated, and their help in developing and critiquing material in the chapters. I am also grateful for the challenge of those who did not welcome this change in me.

Everyone needs an editor, and I have been blessed with the professional services of Lynn Walzer who lovingly volunteered to prepare the manuscript to send to the editors of Findhorn Press. I warmly thank Sabine Weeke at Findhorn for first believing in this project and then shepherding it through the approval and publishing process.

FOREWORD

Gabrielle Chavez has written a book that has touched me deeply. I felt her genuine honesty from the first pages to the last. While reading her book I constantly felt the special presence of a caring person, almost like a loving mother. Gabrielle created a book that inspires not only novices, but people like myself, who have studied dozens of raw recipe books, taught hundreds of classes and written and published several books about raw food.

If I had the chance to start a raw life from the very beginning again and could choose only one book, I would choose Gabrielle's book because it is like an encyclopedia of raw living. *The Raw Food Gourmet* is saturated with countless tips and clever guidelines. Gabrielle clearly explains even the most difficult topics and recipes with her sensible tone. I enjoy Gabrielle's ability to explain complex subjects by illustrating them with brief, well-recognized anecdotes from her own everyday life.

I was especially moved by the strong connection that the author was able to build between healthy eating and spirituality. I find her comments to be brave and honest. For example Gabrielle says: "these reflections on my experience might be useful to health seekers who are also spiritually inclined or ready to take their search for physical vitality to another level." She takes raw food seriously. No kidding! Like any truth in our life, raw food deserves everyone's attention and devotion.

This book is enriched with valuable chapters such as: Long Stays Far From Home, International Travel, Camping and Hiking, Airplanes and Airports, Business Trips and Conventions, Traveling Raw and others.

I want readers to know that my friend Gabrielle is someone who is always smiling. Even when she is not physically smiling, the feeling of a soft smile is shining through her entire being. I get the same easy feeling of a soft smile when I read Gabrielle's book, as when I am actually with her.

Filled with sincere stories, charming humor, and great recipes, *The Raw Food Gourmet* is a gift to humanity that will inspire people all over the world to become healthier.

—Victoria Boutenko, author of *Raw Family : A True Story of Awakening* and *12 Steps to Raw Foods: How to End Your Addiction to Cooked Food*

INTRODUCTION

This book is a way into raw food for the curious along the path I traveled. Going raw is an adventure because even though to many of us it seems intuitively to be the best way to eat, a raw food lifestyle is still profoundly counter-cultural. Successfully staying raw requires a zest for learning not just new foods and methods of preparation, but new ways of relating to food emotionally, mentally, spiritually and socially. Of all the changes of any kind that I've made in a lifetime of change, making the transition to raw only was by far the most radical.

Since experiencing Adelle Davis's *Let's Eat Right to Keep Fit* as a kind of dietary awakening at age 16, I have been fascinated by the stream of information available about healthy food. As a result, I have made many changes in my eating habits.

First, I tried all kinds of "health food" especially what is affectionately known as "health food junk food" which promised both virtue and self-indulgence. In my late 20s I stopped eating meat. When I became a mother, I learned about food allergies and the relationship between a sugar-charged diet, yeast imbalances, antibiotics, and upper respiratory and ear infections. Discovering that I could eliminate problems in my children and myself through food choices was quite empowering.

Because I loved eating and serving food that was soul-satisfying as well as healthy, my cuisine never became ascetic or purist. By age 48, I was in a comfortable groove. I enjoyed the world of ethnic vegetarian dishes when eating out and when creating delectable meals at home for my family and the monthly potlucks of my spiritual healing community. With my husband, Thomas, a former chef who shared my love for rich vegetarian food, and the availability of organic milk, butter, and fine cheeses in our blessed corner of the world, I had settled onto a plateau of being a contented ovo-lacto-vegetarian seemingly for the rest of my life.

A few years earlier I had noticed Jim, a thin, Jesus-lookalike member of our Body Electronics hands-on healing group who always brought some variant of a kale or cabbage salad to community potlucks. He let on that he was a raw-fooder, that is, a person who eats only raw foods. For Jim's sake, I began providing some kind of fruit or raw garden produce along with the cooked dishes we offered. He was quietly grateful and never drew attention to his preferences, even though the healing work we were doing recommended a diet at least 70% raw since it depended on enzymes to be effective at the physical level.

Jim impressed me. When it was his turn to receive hands-on healing from the group, the energy flowing through our fingers to him ignited instantly and burned brightly. When several other young raw fooders joined us, I decided to investigate this new diet by attending one of the International Raw and Living Food Festivals held in the Portland, Oregon, area each year.

Raw food, of course, is not a new diet, but the original way of eating for humans and the ongoing diet for all non-domesticated animals. One argument for raw is simply that, for millions of years until the discovery of fire, our animal bodies evolved on it. Cooking changes food in ways that stress our systems. Proof of this is a well-documented immune reaction—an increase in the white blood cell count that follows cooked (but not raw) meals.

Raw food as a health-conscious choice made its appearance in the 1960s and 1970s when some fruitarians and wheatgrass advocates received notoriety. However, many who tried to follow them didn't succeed because unadorned raw vegetables failed to satisfy most of us. That was then. The new, raw food diet I will share with you in this book is called "Raw Gourmet."

Raw gourmet food was a revelation to me. Most everything I sampled at the festival was both utterly healthy and surprised me by tasting great. The food also had an almost spiritual quality—one that I can only describe as "aliveness." Beyond that, the diversity of foods and preparations presented was amazing. Unlike traditional cuisines such as French, Chinese or Middle Eastern, raw gourmet is still evolving and exploding creatively. So as well as taking in the lectures on the various benefits of going raw, I attended food demonstrations and classes led by brilliant young chefs as well as already established raw culinary celebrities.

I noticed that those festival attendees who were devotees of an extreme raw diet fell into roughly two categories: people who were desperately ill and searching for a miracle (who looked pretty terrible) and those who were on a health food adventure and had found this to be the best choice yet. Many of these persons displayed boundless energy and an intriguing psychic clarity. Inspired by that week, Thomas bought me my first gourmet "uncook" book and we began to eat more fresh and raw food along with our Fettuccine Alfredo and designer chocolate brownies.

It took us a full year until the next festival to take the 100% plunge. Actually I had been convinced by what I learned the first year and decided to wait for him since sharing food practically defines family. It is wise advice for those who choose to go all raw to be gentle like our friend Jim, not judging or criticizing the way others eat. I never let myself forget that I happily ate cooked food well into maturity. Rather than attack anyone's eating habits or beliefs, I wish to appeal to your reason and taste buds.

Of vital assistance to our success was the support of others who had also elected to swim against the tide to make such an enormous change at so many levels from theory to practice in their daily personal and social lives. If you decide to go down this path, look around for your fellow travelers. Search the internet for raw food classes, resources, vacations and the like, and ask locally at co-ops and other places that sell health food for contacts, restaurants and potlucks. Start your own support and learning group by inviting health-conscious friends and family to a raw-themed party.

There are many people who are interested in more physical or spiritual vitality or who share your ecological values. These people will walk with you, at least part way, becoming a source of encouragement rather than criticism for your positive lifestyle changes. Some will even try your new foods and admit they taste pretty good. Jim says, "Acknowledge that you are a pioneer, and applaud yourself, even if no one else does. Pioneers by definition are not part of the pack."

I found, to my great joy, that the benefits of eating more living foods quickly become apparent. Like water on a parched desert, my body welcomed the new enzymes and nutrients the raw food was making available. For me the rewards came the very first week with a noticeable increase in energy and a spiritual awareness akin to what I had only experienced previously during fasts. Eating this way since early 2001, these and other benefits have continued, creating a positive feedback cycle.

A word about sudden transitions from a mostly cooked diet to 100% raw: I say, go for it if you are convinced and can marshal the resources to succeed as we did. But expect your body to respond dramatically. The energy added to your system might be used to initiate a major detoxification. Initially, both of us lost a large amount of weight as our physiques adjusted to the sudden change. You can easily avoid alarming your friends and family by a more phased-in transition if you wish. Even if it takes years to make a full transition, every choice made to eat food raw instead of cooked is a life-giving gain.

In our exploration of this lifestyle, we discovered a world of complex and sometimes contradictory food beliefs within the raw community. Raw purists may disdain anything from the use of condiments and dehydrators in raw gourmet food to combining certain fruits and vegetables in one meal or eating any grains, nuts or legumes at all. As I've listened to them, I've realized these dogmas were developed for folks who had already destroyed their digestion or who had specific health issues. Figure out what works for you.

To succeed in my transition, I gave myself permission to eat anything I wanted, whenever I wanted, in whatever quantity I wanted, as long as it was still a raw or living food. (Living foods are those which may have been processed by fermenting, freezing, drying or blending but not to the point of killing all the enzymes.) That approach has worked for me. Everyone is different and there is the beauty of choice and learning. The best advice I got when I started was to listen to my own biofeedback system, notice how I felt after I ate, and adjust accordingly.

This biofeedback mechanism works especially well if you have been fully raw for six months or more and then suddenly binge on a big cooked meal. Ouch. Or so I've been told. I've kept myself so satisfied with raw gourmet food that I've never reverted to cooked food.

It appears that the better persons have cared for themselves (or the younger they are) the more they can enjoy the full spectrum of raw gourmet dishes and not have to be concerned with draconian raw rescue diets. But whatever your condition, be of good cheer. Eating raw will improve your health. Wheatgrass juice and elimination diets will always be an option if you need them. But if you'd like to have your cake and eat it, too, raw gourmet is the way to go.

CHAPTER 1

RAW CURIOUS

Thank you for picking up this book. Perhaps you are intrigued with the idea that "gourmet raw" not only might be a very healthy diet, but it also might be satisfying and fun. For me, this is the essence of gourmet raw food. It does not deprive you, but enhances vitality while providing pleasurable, satisfying eating.

Perhaps someone who loves you wants you to consider including more living enzymes in your diet. Please forgive me if I seem pushy in my enthusiasm. And thank you for your tolerance which helps keep my zeal in perspective.

Perhaps you are responsible for feeding children and other loved ones and you wish to learn a better way. As a meal provider, I want to offer the best I know to those I feed. I never could be content to serve food I believed was unhealthy, even as my views changed.

Perhaps you need to cure some specific condition and you wonder if this could help. Yes, many have cured "terminal" cancer and other "incurable" chronic diseases with a living foods diet, especially raw vegetable juices. Going raw will give your body the foundation to stop degenerating and even regenerate. I wish I had known this sooner, but am grateful I came across it before it was a desperate choice.

Perhaps you are interested in spiritual growth and practice. For reasons I will discuss in the chapter "Raw Spirituality," one of the great benefits of not eating cooked food appears to be a greater facility of concentration, prayer, and meditation.

Perhaps you are passionately committed to caring for the earth and willing to make a significant personal commitment to reducing pollution and global warming. When I went raw, the amount of non-recyclable trash and packaging waste I generated suddenly became miniscule. I began purchasing in bulk, directly from farmers as much as possible and growing more food myself. I also had the energy and desire to walk more and drive less. Raw fooders eat low on the food chain and support sustainable and organic agriculture.

So, if you answer "Yes" to any of the following:

- You are a lover of food
- You are a lover of life
- You are a lover of others
- You are a lover of spirit
- You are a lover of the earth

Then I invite you to keep reading.

WHY "NOT RAW"

Here are the common concerns and criticisms you might hear as you consider a raw lifestyle, and some useful responses:

• Where will I get my protein?

Protein is everywhere in food. It is what gives food its shape. Many of us have been brainwashed to believe that the best source, even the only source, of those amino acids in protein which are essential to our bodies is from (cooked) meat and other animal products. In fact, heating protein even to the temperature that coddles eggs, denatures it and makes some of the essential amino acids unavailable to the body to assimilate. Microwaving, which may raise the internal temperature of food to 2000 degrees, is even more degrading to the molecular structure of proteins, altering some beyond recognition to our systems or leaving behind only damaged proteins with which to build muscle and other tissue. Carnivores who eat concentrated animal proteins may have better survival odds than cooked food vegans. But "raw fooders" get quality protein from everything they eat and assimilate those proteins far better than persons who cook all their meat and vegetables.

Eating food uncooked preserves the enzymes (which are also protein) that are vital to digestion and assimilation. This frees the pancreas from diverting energy to produce enzymes for digestion and allows it to do its main job of producing systemic enzymes to support the internal protein metabolism and catabolism processes of a healthy body.

You could gently suggest to those who are concerned about protein that they might rather ask where they are getting their enzymes—packaged free with their food, or at significant cost to their overworked pancreases?

• It's too much trouble.

Going raw can be as simple as peeling bananas, rinsing carrots, and eating nuts and raisins out of a bag. If one of your meals each day is fresh fruit and another is salads, you are already 2/3 raw with very little trouble. Remember, nobody is making you do this or go all the way all at once. Noticing what you already like to eat that can either be consumed uncooked or increased in your diet is an easy way to begin. From time to time, when you would be going to some trouble anyway to make a nice meal for yourself or others, try out some raw recipes and gradually increase the list of things you like to eat. Incrementally add the equipment and staples to your kitchen that make it easy to produce raw gourmet dishes at a moment's notice.

Or, jump in like I did with both feet when you're good and ready and never look back. Then the amount of time and effort needed to master the learning curve will be a welcome part of the adventure.

• It's too expensive.

If you depend on a raw gourmet caterer or restaurant to provide your meals—and if you are lucky enough to have that option—it can be quite expensive, like any fine dining. But if you learn to prepare it yourself, you will be surprised at how much less you spend on food that is likely far superior in quality and variety to how you ate before. In our household, food costs initially dropped 1/3 and eventually to less than one half of what we previously spent as we discovered local growers and began to buy in bulk. A gourmet raw diet saves by avoiding value-added, manufactured items including junk foods and drinks.

Keep in mind the hidden costs of the apparently cheaper processed foods at the fast food drive through or in your neighbor's grocery cart compared to the clutch of avocados in yours. They include processing, packaging, storage, advertising, transportation from farm to factory to store, and all the attendant pollution to name the obvious ones. Then add the health care costs of obesity and other diet-related illnesses. Now the question becomes, "...expensive for whom?"

• It's too time-consuming.

How much time do you currently spend shopping for food, cooking it, or going out to eat? If I go to the supermarket, I head straight for the produce section and then the checkout. I still marvel at how irrelevant the rest of the store is to me now and how fast I can get away from the shopping trance.

Consider that another huge benefit in terms of time that most 100% raw fooders report is less need for sleep. That makes sense as the enzyme-filled food you're eating doesn't overwork your digestion or stress your immune system. After a big cooked dinner, I was always ready for a nap, and needed 8-9 hours of sleep at night to feel refreshed. Now I wake without an alarm, feeling good with 5-7 hours. After a big raw feast, I am energized, not groaning and loosening my belt.

How much time you take to make the transition to a raw lifestyle and then live it is both a learning curve and a matter of personal choice. When my husband and I jumped in, we invested time and money in learning why and how to eat this way. For me it was like taking a university level course to educate and re-educate myself to this diet. Now we are pros at feeding ourselves and others the gourmet raw way from quite simple meals to elaborate feasts. I have more than once prepared and decorated beautiful, tasty, fruit, flower and nut cakes ready to serve in fifteen minutes.

• Isn't raw food more likely to be contaminated with bacteria, such as E. coli?

The main reason that traditional Indian and Chinese cuisine is completely cooked is the unfortunate practice, mostly in the past, of fertilizing fields and gardens with "night soil"—fresh human feces. Cooking was essential then to reduce bacteria and parasite infection. E. coli contamination in our food supply today comes from the poor hygiene practices of food handlers. Interestingly, by far most of the problems have been in animal products and processed foods, although commercial alfalfa sprouts, salad bars, and some produce have been implicated. At-risk populations need to take special care to find clean sources of raw food and wash it well. If I were still eating meat and processed foods, I'd consider myself at risk. But as a raw fooder, my immune system is better than ever and I now know a lot more about where my food is coming from.

On the other hand, over-washing produce is now being recognized as a problem. There are many beneficial microorganisms in the soil, which act as probiotics in our digestive tract, that we are deprived of when we sterilize our food to an unnatural degree. Personally, I'm much more concerned about the pesticides', fungicides', and genetically-modified organisms' (GMOs) interference with my food than some dirt and insects.

As you experience the greater sensitivity to life energy that comes with a raw diet, you can put your awareness to use in choosing food by its aura or intuitive feel, facing a produce bin with the question, what is best? Enjoy the increased fearlessness you will gain with food choices. I do!

• I'd have to give up cheese.

I sympathize if this is an obstacle for you. Before I went raw, I had been a "cheesetarian" for decades. I love cheese. It's the great lacto-vegetarian fast food. For the first six months after going raw, I dreamed about cheese. However, I already knew it wasn't that good for me, especially in the quantities I was consuming it. I had tried to go dairy-free previously, but couldn't overcome my cravings until I went raw. Then I was pleasantly surprised that I managed my cravings without much effort. Now when I'm around it, I remember all the cheese I used to enjoy, give thanks, acknowledge any remaining longing, and realize that I don't want to pay the price in decreased vitality of a mucus-clogged system. The moment passes and the temptation is gone. You do have some choices here. It may be possible to find clean and safe raw cow or goat dairy products, including cheese. If you can get them, that might be an improvement over the pasteurized, homogenized, aseptically packaged, bovine-growth hormone products commonly available. But nearly all people who jump to raw, including myself, also jump to vegan if they weren't already there. Why? At a conference I saw some dark field microscopy slides of the blood of people who consumed raw dairy foods, that showed evidence of parasites absent in the blood of raw vegans. And the increased sensitivity that grew from eating all raw has made cheese and the whole dairy production industry that delivers it to me more difficult for my conscience, as well as my digestion, to stomach.

That said, there are versions of raw vegan cheese you can concoct with nut and seed milks. In most cases, I won't pretend they taste very much like my formerly beloved dairy cheeses and they don't hold the same place in my diet as cheese used to. I accept this as a blessing, not a problem. And I'll always have my fond memories to look back upon.

• If I don't eat cheese or dairy products, where do I get my calcium?

Much of this concern is the result of the relentless misinformation campaign of the milk industry. While dairy products might have more total milligrams of calcium than plant foods, along with meat they also have large amounts of phosphorus. The more phosphorus ingested, the more calcium is needed to maintain a proper blood pH. Therefore, drinking milk and eating cheese will result in a net calcium loss for the body. Our bodies do need a variety of calcium salts, so supplementation could provide this if that is your choice and your need. But they are also in the green leafy vegetables, especially bio-available in juiced form, for those of us who don't chew well.

• If I don't eat meat, where do I get my B-12?

Here a debate does rage within the raw community. Supplementation is a simple option for vegans who feel the need or show symptoms of a deficiency. Our experience is, that a varied gourmet raw diet, including fermented foods such as sauerkraut and kefir which feed and repopulate the colonies of bacteria in the gut that produce B-12 and other B vitamins, makes this unnecessary. Sea vegetables, algae such as spirulina and chlorella, and bee pollen, especially pre-digested in kefir, are also possible sources of B-12 for those who don't want to consume meat, eggs or dairy—raw or cooked. Nutritional yeast, a by-product of brewing loaded with B vitamins, also provides B-12, though it is not raw.

• I'd be hungry.

This is an important consideration because feeling hungry and unsatisfied will cause you to yield to the ever-present temptation to grab what everyone else eats. The first thing to realize is that you aren't necessarily hungry on a raw diet because your body needs nutrition. It's more likely to be habit, expectation, and cravings that are bothering you. These will all pass as your new lifestyle replaces the old, but in the meantime, anticipate this challenge and make it easy on yourself. Don't let yourself get hungry without raw food in reach. Always have access to pure drinking water and try that first. Thirst signals can be misinterpreted as hunger pangs. I used to keep trail mix and "Crunchies" (see p. 77) in our car at all times. Our refrigerator typically contains several kinds of fresh whole fruit, raw almond butter, celery and carrots for snacking. I keep jars of flax crackers, dried bananas, prunes, and raw cookies on my counter to eat when hunger strikes or to fill a baggie and take with me to work. The great thing is you don't have to feel guilty no matter how much of these treats you consume. You could live on them.

• How do you maintain a healthy weight when all you eat is fruits and vegetables?

I wish you could see Thomas. He eats much less than I do, but remains "substantial." That's true of some 100% raw fooders, but not most. Most lose weight and stay fairly thin effortlessly. We consider that one of the benefits! If you jump in "cold turkey" like we did, expect to lose weight, especially at first. I lost 20 pounds and went from a size 12 to a 6 for a few months. This is because a dramatic change in eating habits takes some time to adjust to physically and in relearning how to nourish yourself. I admit I looked somewhat wasted that first summer, but I still felt great. By the end of the year, I had regained the 20 pounds but was only a size 8—and have been ever since. With a raw energy lifestyle, I never have to worry about my weight, one way or another. How you respond will have a lot to do with your genetic predisposition and metabolism. Raw food choices that tend to put weight on are a preponderance of nut milks, smoothies, fruits and other sweets with less of the balancing plant chlorophyll—green foods. It's not too hard to figure out what you need. Listen to your own body.

• It's lonely.

Yes, eating is a social pursuit and so very much of our socializing involves food. Eating together bonds families, ethnic groups, and religions. Eating separate or apart can severely challenge those ties. Ten years into my first marriage, my then husband, two children and myself were all on different diets for various reasons. He liked the Standard American Diet of his childhood, with an emphasis on beef and pork products. I strove to provide our first child with what I then considered to be healthy alternatives. Our youngest child was born with food allergies and an autoimmune disease that were well managed with an elimination diet—eliminating wheat, dairy, refined sugar, yeast, and all processed foods and chemicals. I was an ovo-lacto-vegetarian. Catering four different meals each day and policing my children's choices when their father tempted them by example or offer was stressful for me and exacerbated the tensions in our family every time we sat down to eat. Although that didn't end our marriage, it didn't help.

Years later, when I met Thomas and discovered he had been a vegetarian longer than I, I knew we had a vital building block for our developing relationship. We were both interested in health, and he was the first to introduce me to the benefits of a raw diet for physical health and a type of healing energy work he practiced called Body Electronics. However, he had twice tried and failed to go raw because the regimen presented to him then—wheatgrass, sprouts and plain vegetables—felt boring and unsatisfying. Convinced in theory, but not quite in practice, we began swallowing a couple of tablets of food enzymes with our luscious, cheesy meals to compensate for our cooked food choices.

During our second year of attending the International Raw and Living Food Festival, we made friends with the "Raw Family," Igor, Victoria, Sergei, and Valya Boutenko, who blessed us with platters of their beautiful raw food three times a day. By the end of the week, Thomas was thinking that maybe he could eat raw—gourmet raw. Attending a final presentation by Victoria provided the rationale to go along with the tasty food. Victoria showed a video of two persons' blood, a cooked food vegan and a meat eater, both of whom had gone all raw for six weeks, clearly showing their red blood cells floating like flying saucers the way a newborn baby's red blood cells might appear. A trained homeopath, Thomas recognized this as most unusual. Then she showed the video of their blood six hours after the meat eater had broken his raw fast with a chicken wing and the vegan had broken her fast with a bit of baked potato. The red blood cells were clumped together like stacks of pancakes as seen in "normal" adult blood. Thomas knew that he had just seen another reason why raw fooders have more energy besides enzyme availability: the red blood cells, whose job is to conduct oxygen to the vital organs, were able to move freely.

Victoria closed the sale by discussing her research indicating that eating cooked food is actually an addiction; that is, an unnatural, unhealthy behavior which, once engaged, becomes a vicious cycle of craving what is not good for you. She postulated that craving cooked food might even be the original addiction underlying all subsequent addictions. No other animal cooks its food or thinks it needs to. Breast-fed infants universally spit out the first offerings of cooked gruel until, with it shoved in their faces again and again by loving parents, they give up and the addiction cycle begins. Victoria insisted that it is actually easier to go 100% raw than almost all raw. Imagine trying to succeed in being 5-15% alcoholic.

Thomas came back from that lecture and announced to me: "I'm going 100% raw." I said, "OK, then I'll join you, because you can't do it alone." We haven't looked back since.

Frankly, the social aspect of eating raw is still the most challenging for me. Not everyone I know is interested in my lifestyle and some feel threatened or judged by it. Food shame and guilt are still big parts of our culture. Go easy on your friends and relations. Affirm that for you the relationship is more important than the food you eat or don't eat together.

When I came back from my "conversion" at the Raw and Living Foods Festival, I told my 18-year-old son who was still living with us and had been enduring our vegetarianism, "There is too big a gap between the way I am going to eat now and the way you want to eat. Let's make a deal. I'll take you to the grocery store and buy whatever you want that isn't junk food on two conditions: you cook it and you clean it up."

He was overjoyed and we could still sit down at the table together with mutual acceptance. Eventually I was willing to cook some of his favorite comfort foods for him and he was willing to try some of my treats and award me grudging respect.

My raw friends share these suggestions to make the social part of eating raw easier:

- Be prepared to talk about it, but notice when to stop.

- Evangelize and win your friends over by being willing to bring extra treats to share with them. Then your discoveries can become a source of interest and unity, not division.

• If your friends and family hesitate to invite you over because they think they can't feed you, swear you're happy with just salad, or offer to bring a special dish you can eat to contribute to the feast. After all, nearly everyone can eat your food, and there is an increasing number of lactose-gluten-carbo-or-whatever-intolerant folk who will be grateful to you and, incidentally, make your peculiarity seem less conspicuous.

When I go out to eat, it's not for the food but the company. Unless it's a raw restaurant, I either don't go hungry or bring an avocado to enhance the house salad. See the chapter "Traveling Raw" for more tips. On the plus side, I regularly host and participate in raw potlucks which have become a fun new part of our social calendar. I have also learned that bringing exceptionally appealing raw gourmet finger foods, salads, and desserts to social gatherings is a great way to participate in "breaking bread together," as well as share the treasure I have found with others.

"WHY NOT RAW?"

I didn't realize it at the time, but going 100% raw was the largest, most thorough change I had ever made in my life—impacting everything I did for personal and planetary transformation. In changing the way I ate, I had to learn new things, meet new people, and think new thoughts. It changed the way I shopped and spent my time. Being successfully raw changed how I felt about myself and my self development. I became more sensitive to energy and more masterful applying it in healing modalities. My vitality and enthusiasm for life and work increased markedly. Now I feel an empowering alignment between my core values and lifestyle choices that I never experienced before. Given these many benefits, I would recommend considering a raw and living foods lifestyle because it:

• Supports overall healing. Raw fooders find that nagging chronic problems from acne, allergies, dandruff, post-nasal drip, constipation, high blood pressure, depression, backaches, frequent infections, pre-menstrual symptoms, obesity and the like just disappear.

Cancer, heart disease and many other life-threatening conditions can either be prevented or cured with a raw diet.

• Provides more energy.

• Avoids all the chemicals added and nutrients lost in processed (cooked) food.

• Is far less costly on a personal as well as on a planetary scale to eat this way.

• Puts you at peace with your own body.

• Puts you at peace with the animal kingdom.

• Develops your relationship with and appreciation of the plant kingdom.

• Is the missing piece in being a successful healthy vegan.

• Offers a way to be congruent with your ecological values and health beliefs.

• Is a way to love and care for yourself.

• Is an effective means to free yourself from addictions and, thus, increase self esteem.

• Supports spiritual practice.

• Raises and clarifies awareness of energy and increases capacity to be a channel of energy and spirit.

• Heightens the sensitivity of your taste buds and your potential pleasure in food.

• Allows for creativity and self expression through the art of food preparation.

• Is a radical personal and political commitment for a better world.

• Includes raw chocolate. It wasn't available when we first went raw, so count your blessings!

CHAPTER 2

THE ART OF RAW GOURMET

I'll admit it. Raw gourmet food "gilds the lily." Little that we can do to plain raw fruits, seeds, nuts and vegetables will improve their nutritional gift to us. Yet all of us who have grown up in a cooked food culture have learned to enjoy and even crave certain flavors, textures, and combinations associated with our past. Most humans demand more of food than simple nutrition; we expect it to give us comfort and pleasure as well.

Chad Sarno, an international raw gourmet chef, tells the story to his classes about leaping into a raw lifestyle upon becoming convinced, as a young man, that fruit and salads were far healthier than the rich Italian food of his heritage. After a period of time, he realized that, while his physical self was very happy and satisfied with that simple diet, his emotional self was unfulfilled, so he went back to home cooking. Still desirous of making the change, he realized that what made food comforting (especially Italian food) was largely the fat and salt content. When he began experimenting with raw gourmet dishes, including liberal amounts of fat and salt, he was able to help himself and many others become successfully raw-gourmet.

Clever raw chefs have discovered that there are many ways to create satisfying variety in taste, texture, and appearance of foods without killing all of the enzymes. Chopping, blending, dehydrating, juicing, fermenting, marinating, sprouting, and using condiments are the major means to this end, replacing boiling, baking, frying, microwaving, and the like. A little information about equipment and processes will help you to become a successful raw gourmet chef.

FOOD DEHYDRATOR

For me this is an essential tool for a joyful, 100% raw lifestyle. Let's clear up right now that dried food is not raw except in the important technical sense that it need not be heated at temperatures resulting in nutrient destruction. This destruction begins at about 105 degrees Fahrenheit and is complete above 140 degrees. My goal is to encompass all of the artistry, pleasure, convenience, and satisfaction gained in cooking food without destroying its nutritional value, and a food dehydrator greatly expands my options for accomplishing this. Owning a food dehydrator also means you can dry anything you make fresh for later consumption.

If you live in a hot, dry place, God's sunshine may do the drying job for you gratis. In the summer, I load trays with sliced plums and tomatoes and put them out on the deck. Alternatively, you can build your own dehydrator, spend hundreds of dollars for a very fine Excalibur 9-tray model, or do what I did my first three years of going raw: find the simple, cheap, round food dryers at garage sales and thrift shops and spend almost nothing. The trade-off is these cheap ones lack a thermostat and sometimes even a fan and may, therefore, heat unevenly from top to bottom depending upon what is being dried and what stage of drying it is in. But with attentiveness to rotating trays, I managed to turn out a constant stream of crackers, breads, brownies, fruit leathers and bars, seed and nut crunchies, "graw-nola" pie crusts, burgers, warm soups and entrees, and much more to keep us from missing any of our former pleasures.

After three years, I did some research and replaced my Roncos with a neat little 6-tray L'Equip, complete with fan and thermostat. It is smaller than an Excalibur and still has a hole in the middle of the rectangular trays so it doesn't make big sheets of crackers, but it is also much less expensive for the features I need while still large enough to dry a gallon of graw-nola all at once. Search the internet for the best prices. You'll find used dehydrators for sale on eBay as well.

KNIVES

Any chef, cooked or raw, will tell you to invest in at least one high quality knife that feels good in your hand. It will greatly increase your pleasure and speed in food preparation and stand you in good stead when a food processor might not be available. Keep it sharp. A mandoline or v-slicer is a great accessory gadget for paper-thin slices and julienne noodles and is faster and more accurate than most of us knife-wielding amateurs. Consider other miscellaneous slicing gadgets, especially vegetable spiralizers, that can turn a few zucchinis into a bowl of noodles in moments.

FOOD PROCESSOR

In my stove-retired lifestyle, the food processor has become my stove, that is, the machine I use most in food preparation. Raw recipes frequently speak of employing an "S" blade, although the shredding wheel is also great for preparing large quantities of cabbage for sauerkraut.

Unfortunately, raw cuisine seems to be hard on home-grade food processors. We quickly stripped the gears of the one we already owned with our early raw experiments and then replaced it with a brand new Cuisinart that didn't last much longer. Our problems don't come with the motors, but the blades which dull quickly, and the plastic parts, especially the safety locking mechanism without which the machine will not work. Discovering that replacement parts might be half the cost of a new processor, we turned to thrift shops and garage sales, where we have been able to acquire hand-me-down processors for $20 or less as we needed them.

In the Findhorn community, machines are given names to recognize and honor their place and purpose. I named my first processor Chakra, and the rest are numbered in a lineage like queens and popes. These recipes were developed in my fourth Chakra.

BLENDER

If you already have one of these common appliances, you can make lots of raw recipes right away without buying any more equipment. Nut milks, smoothies, sauces, salad dressings, icings, pestos, and soups are just some of the items you can make using a blender. When you are in a blender buying mode—and you will be soon if you become a raw gourmet, because most of these machines don't hold up to serious regular use—consider finding the means to buy a powerful, high quality one. Unless you are lucky enough to inherit one of these, such as a Vita-Mix or K-Tec, or find one at a garage sale, expect to spend $300-400. A high-speed, industrial blender will pulverize much more thoroughly and not suffer a motor meltdown when you work with thick sauces.

ELECTRIC JUICER

Juicers concentrate the nutrients of plants by separating the blood from the bone, so to speak. Like blenders, they do our chewing for us, and deliver nutrients faster. They also speed up oxidation, so fresh juices should be consumed right away if possible. There's no point in keeping them in the refrigerator for longer than a day, and I wouldn't wait that long. Different juicers offer different technologies which handle some vegetables and fruits better than others. Some, like the Champion-type models with a blank plate, expand gourmet raw possibilities for making easy nut butters and grinding frozen fruit into velvety loops like soft serve ice cream. I have a Champion, but it doesn't do wheatgrass, so I also invested in a Samson, which does. Not everybody needs a mechanical juicer. Take some time to figure out what you will truly use before you make the investment.

NYLON MESH BAG OR CHEESECLOTH

You will need one of these to strain blended ingredients for drinks or nut milks, as well as to make cheese. Purchased or home made mesh or muslin bags are easiest to use, but a large square of double layered cheesecloth held in a colander and then carefully gathered together at the edges to squeeze or drip can do the job, too.

FERMENTING

To make these "living foods," you either use a culture or trust the air. Sauerkraut, for instance, can be so easy and cheap if it works, just shredding cabbage, packing it in a non-metal container with salt, covering it with a weight and eating it a few days later. You can increase the odds that it will work out to your taste by using somebody else's raw sauerkraut as a starter, if available. In my experience, yogurts made from nut or seed milks usually sour fine on the kitchen counter without an added culture.

Rejuvalac is a fermented liquid drink cultured from sprouted grains. To make your own, rinse 1 cup (140g) of any sprouted grain (wheat and rye berries are commonly used) and place in a clean quart (litre) jar with filtered water. Cover the jar with a clean cloth and leave in a warm place. In a few days, you should have a sour, lemony-tasting drink with, perhaps, a little effervescence. If so, strain it off (you can repeat the process with the same grains once or twice more), and then store it in the refrigerator for up to a week. If it doesn't taste sour and a little lemony, and it doesn't smell good, throw it out and start over with new grains and a clean jar. Besides being a healthful and not too bad tasting drink all by itself, rejuvelac is used as a starter for seed and nut cheese.

Our favorite cultured drink is **kefir**, similar to liquid yogurt but with a more complex combination of beneficial probiotics. Cultured for hundreds of years in goat and cow milk, it is also possible to successfully ferment grape juice, coconut water, and nut milks with kefir grains. I drank kefir smoothies every day for the first year of going raw. They greatly helped me feel satisfied and happy during my transition, especially when accompanied with chewy raw cookies, bars, and breads or poured over a bowl of "Graw-nola." See the chapter "Cake for Breakfast" for recipes. These fermented drinks may contain a small percentage of alcohol, but far less than wine—which many also consider a raw food.

Miso and **soy sauce** are two other fermented foods you can buy which expand the flavor possibilities of raw food, although some believe they encourage yeasts in the body and recommend avoiding them. Miso contributes a salty, vaguely cheesy taste to some dishes. Nama Shoyu soy sauce from the Ohsawa company is the only brand I know that is not re-pasteurized after fermenting (thus qualifying it as a living food) and it tastes wonderful.

MARINATING

This means soaking chopped fruits or vegetables in a liquid such as olive oil, soy sauce, lemon juice or vinegar, often flavored with garlic, ginger or other spices for a period of time. Marinades may infuse flavor and/or soften the texture of foods. Acidic marinades, especially with salt added, will break down tough plant fibers such as kale, much as cooking does but without the heat.

SPROUTING

Sprouting renders nuts, seeds, and especially legumes edible. This is partly because sprouting breaks the hard seed casing, but also because the process wakes up the dormant life force and makes it available to digestion. The balance of nutrients also changes as the sprouts green and grow. Most grains and many seeds and legumes, such as garbanzo beans (chick peas), hulled sunflower seeds, buckwheat, and oat groats are best sprouted only a day or two, just until they have little tails. The easiest way to do this is to soak them in water overnight and in the morning pour them into a strainer. Leave them in or near the sink and rinse them once or twice while waiting for the tails to grow before using or storing them in the refrigerator.

One thing I learned after becoming raw was to soak my nuts for at least a few hours, and then rinse them before eating. This washes away the enzyme-inhibiting chemicals nature equips them with to prevent premature spoiling or sprouting. Some people who thought they were allergic to nuts find that nuts are quite digestible after soaking and rinsing, especially deciduous nuts, such as almond, walnuts, hazelnuts, and pecans. Macadamias, cashews, pistachios, and pine nuts are not improved by soaking as far as I can see. I sometimes recommend gently re-drying wet nuts before using them in recipes because it restores the crunch and approaches a toasted flavor.

Certain nuts labeled "raw" such as most cashews and pecans have been boiled or steamed in processing to remove shells and are no longer capable of sprouting since they are now dead. Eat them if you want, but don't kid yourself that they are raw. Sorry. Even though cashews make great icings and other desserts, I have not included them in recipes because truly raw ones are unlikely to be found in stores. You can buy pecans in the shell or order truly raw (and so far, truly much more expensive) cashews and shelled pecans from a reputable raw supplier in order to enjoy these rich, high fat nuts in gourmet raw recipes.

CONDIMENTS

• Salt

Ordinary table salt has been superheated, stripped of its minerals, and loaded with questionable chemical additives. Don't use it. Even most "sea salt" has been heated and bleached. Raw (and other) gourmets use naturally-colored salts that retain their mineral and flavor complexity. Grey Celtic Sea salt is popular. My favorite is a pink salt mined in Utah and marketed as RealSalt. Since it comes from an ancient sea bed, it doesn't contain any of the chemical and radioactive pollution of today's seas.

• Oil

There are a growing number of unrefined, low-temperature, extracted vegetable oils available, but the gold standard is still the universally available extra virgin olive oil. It works fine in all savory dishes. Experiment with raw sesame, hemp, pumpkin seed oil, and the like, if you can find them. For added fat in sweet dishes, use a nut oil, especially unrefined coconut oil which has a wonderful, fresh flavor.

• Vinegar

So far it seems that the only commercially available raw vinegar is apple cider vinegar. All of the others I know of have been pasteurized to stop the fermentation process and standardize the acidity. Too bad. Nevertheless, I still keep balsamic vinegar on hand to flavor the apple cider vinegar in certain dishes. Tiny amounts of non-raw condiments are not going to hurt you even if you have been 100% raw for a long time.

• Extracts and Flavorings

Alcohol and non-alcohol extracts such as vanilla, almond, peppermint, and butterscotch, as well as food grade essential oils including lemon, orange, and lavender, will enhance your raw gourmet creations and help satisfy the longing for remembered flavors. If you can afford it, use vanilla beans instead of extract in blended icings and ice creams for an over-the-top, gourmet raw experience.

• Thickeners

Flax seeds, brown or golden, become a gelatinous mass when soaked in water. Judicious amounts can be used to thicken puddings and sauces. Flax seed meal, which is made by powdering the seeds dry in a blender or grinder, is the secret ingredient holding together many raw "breads." Raw chefs also use psyllium seed husk powder for puddings, pies, and mousses. It's definitely good for your digestion but makes a granulated texture not everyone loves. Agar-agar and carageenan, ingredients used in kosher gelatins which are extracted from seaweed, give a creamier mouth feel but must be dissolved in very hot water first and are not raw. Carageenan in its raw seaweed form called Irish Moss (*Chrondrus crispus*) can be used. Another way to thicken sauces is to incorporate dried foods. Dried tomatoes thicken salsa and marinara sauce beautifully. Dried nuts and mushrooms help condense gravies, mayonnaise, and cream sauces. Dried fruits will thicken pies, puddings, cakes, and sweet sauces. Putting dishes in a dehydrator will drive off moisture. Freezing and partially thawing also works for some desserts.

• Sweeteners

Raw gourmets have many, sweeter choices than refined sugars. Dried fruits, especially raisins, figs, prunes, and dates are good for sweetening desserts. Ripe bananas and coconut can lend sweetness to a dish. I like raw honey, but that makes me a "bee-gan," not a pure vegan. Raw agave nectar, with many of the same culinary properties and a mild taste, is now available and can be used like honey. Other vegan options include maple syrup—definitely not raw—and evaporated sugar cane juice marketed as Rapadura. Another sweetener I use whenever possible is *Stevia rebaudiana*, a little green plant native to South America with very sweet tasting leaves but no sugar molecules in any form. Interestingly, as an herb it is used to feed and heal the pancreas, which is often damaged by refined sugar consumption. The powdered leaves are 30 times as sweet-tasting as sugar, and the white powder extract is 200 times sweeter. Do not shake the stevia bottle over your dish unless you have faultless coordination! I use it in small amounts in most desserts to lessen the need for other sweeteners, but not so much that the licorice aftertaste is detectable. Speaking of licorice, the root powder also works as a mild sweetener if you like the flavor.

• Herbs and Spices

These are the glory of gourmet raw cuisine. Raw restaurateur Juliano says, "Always take the spices to the edge!" You don't have to go as far as he does to create amazing flavors in your raw food. Employing the same spices used in ethnic dishes allows gourmet raw chefs to come up with "copycat" dishes like raw lasagna, pad Thai, hummus, curries, and the like that taste quite similar to the old favorites and, in many cases, much better.

Use most spices in powdered form. Owning an inexpensive coffee bean/spice grinder to process whole spices allows you to fill your nostrils, heart, and kitchen with the aromatherapy of the just-released fragrance of cinnamon, chocolate, cumin, dried orange peel, and the like. Store-bought powders work just fine as long as they have not been sitting half-used in a metal container since the 1950s in the back of your spice cupboard. Please shake the contents of all such artifacts onto your compost heap and, thereafter, mercifully return any accumulated herbs and spices to mother earth after a year.

I use fresh herbs whenever possible, especially ginger, garlic, basil, oregano, parsley, cilantro (coriander leaf), thyme, fennel, sage and mint. See the chapter "Gardening in the Raw" for ways to keep most of these on hand year-round.

TIPS FOR THE RAW CHEF

Working with raw recipes invites both a sense of artistry and adventure. Whole natural foods are not standardized. No two lemons are quite the same in amount of juice or acidity. Tomatoes have moods. Weather makes a difference. Different crops of fruits and nuts express their own vintages. Personal tastes vary. Therefore, approach recipes as experiments, adjusting amounts and making substitutions as you please. In most cases, this will not interfere with the results the way it does in cooking, because without added heat, we are doing very little food chemistry. The bright flavors and aromas of raw gourmet food offer themselves to your palate one after another, not depleted and melted together like common cooking.

Be aware that the quality of your raw materials and the quality of your added love will determine the excellence of your final result. The fresher, more local, more organic, and sustainably grown the better. Your own awakening taste buds and palate will surely guide you to choose the finest ingredients available. Then take the best you can gather and suffuse it with heart as you prepare and serve your blessed food.

As you interact more and more with these naked flavors, a growing attunement and confidence can free you from measuring cups and spoons altogether, allowing you to prepare wonderful dishes by sight, taste, flavor memory, and feel. Play with the condiments, adding more salt, oil, sweet, sour, or spicy notes until it tastes good. Give yourself permission to fail and make a compost offering if it doesn't. Not every experiment is a guaranteed success.

CHAPTER 3

GLOBAL FRUIT

I used to think avocados were a luxury food, and had only tasted the smelly but ambrosial durian fruit once on a trip to the Philippines. Upon entering the raw world, avocados suddenly became an affordable staple and durians an excuse for a party. Part of the fun and benefit of a raw lifestyle for me has been discovering the wide diversity of foods I can learn how to eat. Current United States government dietary guidelines recommend nine servings each day of fruits and vegetables for each of us. Raw fooders needn't be concerned.

Following is a quick introduction to my favorite raw food friends which appear in the recipes in this book.

• Avocado

Avocados are available fresh and good in all seasons because they ripen off the tree. This also means you can buy them green and unripened to take on trips and time their ripening to your needs. Even most conventional recipes feature avocados raw because they taste best that way. With their portability, ease of eating, all eight essential amino acids, a taste almost everyone likes, and a satisfying, healthy fat content, avocados are the friend of both beginning and seasoned raw fooders. You could live on them just plain. Feed them to babies. Simply spread their creamy flesh on romaine lettuce leaves with sprouts and a slice of tomato, roll up and feast. Or enjoy them in more elaborate recipes. The first year we went raw, Thomas and I could go through two dozen avocados in just a week. Even now, there are always some in our refrigerator.

• Carob

Carob is the long, wide bean of a type of locust tree which grows in warm climates. It is somewhat sweet with a taste and color reminiscent of chocolate, to which it is not related. Another name for carob is Saint John's Bread, a reference to its being half the diet of John the Baptist, of biblical fame, who was said to live on "locusts and honey." Looks to me like this famous ascetic had a major sweet tooth.

Since, along with its other virtues, carob has no caffeine, it has long been used as a chocolate substitute. Raw gourmets have found several ways to make carob taste more like chocolate in recipes, although its own native caramel-like flavor is just fine with many folk. Vanilla helps, as does the addition of powdered orange or tangerine peel which add some complexity and bitter notes. Surprisingly, a tiny amount of cayenne can do the same thing. I said tiny. Other ways to fool chocoholics are to add the strong flavors of cinnamon or peppermint to it. It looks so much like the chocolate people are expecting, that many don't notice it isn't.

Carob is usually sold as a powder. The powder is almost always roasted to extend shelf life. You can order raw carob powder through your health food store if you ask for it specifically, or from the online raw food web sites, of which there are a growing number. I have also ground the whole dried pods in a blender.

• Chocolate

I thought I had to give up chocolate along with cheese when I went raw, and for three years I managed perfectly well with carob. Then, like the grace of God, some entrepreneurial raw fooders succeeded in bringing organic raw chocolate nibs, or beans, from Ecuador to market. At first only unpeeled beans were available, and Thomas once spent three hours lovingly rubbing the tight skins off half a pound of beans so I could make a real raw chocolate cake. Now you can buy peeled nibs for the same price—which is not cheap.

These same entrepreneurs are now insisting that chocolate really is good for you, at least raw chocolate, citing its high magnesium content and natural endorphin effect. I surely want to believe them.

I don't know if there are any culinary reasons why chocolate beans are roasted, because the raw ones taste just the same. To use them like cocoa powder in recipes, grind the peeled beans as fine as your equipment allows. Whole beans can be tossed in a blender with nut milk, sweetener, vanilla, and a ripe frozen banana for a raw chocolate shake.

I have noticed that it helps to substitute a little carob powder for some of the raw chocolate if the dark color is important to your final result. This also cuts some of the cost.

• **Coconut**

As a little girl, I thought I hated coconut. But I had never tasted it fresh.

Fresh coconuts are available in at least three forms:

> • The most familiar mature coconut sold husked in the whole brown shell.

> • A less mature version, found especially in Asian markets, with a white shell.

> • The green or young coconut, sometimes called Thai young coconut, sold with most of the white husk still attached that you need a machete or cleaver to open.

Each has different uses and value in raw cuisine. The mature, brown coconuts can be cracked with a hammer, separated from the shell, sliced, and then grated with the peel on in a food processor. It can be used in recipes or dried for later use. Make sure it looks, tastes, and smells good before you use it. The meat might still be salvageable if the water is rancid. Many supermarket managers mistakenly believe that coconuts last forever in produce bins and might sell you one that has gone bad inside. Return it and educate them. Or buy your coconuts from markets which serve people from coconut-producing climes. This is less of a problem with white coconuts because they are usually refrigerated.

The younger the coconut, the softer the meat and the less of it which has congealed from the vitamin and mineral packed plasma inside. The youngest coconuts are esteemed for the mildly sweet liquor inside, with any pudding-like meat clinging to the inside of the shell considered a bonus.

Raw gourmets lift the soft meat from split open young coconuts with an upside-down teaspoon, eat "as is" or slice it into thin noodles for Asian-inspired dishes.

To make coconut milk, combine the water inside with the meat in a blender and liquefy it. This can be the basis for soups, smoothies, or rich ice cream. The older the coconut, the thicker the milk will be, but also possibly the grittier, depending on the power of your blender. Straining is a good idea in this case.

Nutritionally, a fresh, whole coconut with its water not only tastes good, but it is also a wonder food. Not only has the saturated fat in coconuts been cleared of guilt, a major constituent of the oil, caprylic acid, has been shown to have powerful anti-viral and anti-fungal effects. When buying coconut oil, make the effort to find a cold-pressed, unrefined version which leaves all of the heavenly taste of the coconut's essential oil intact.

How to Open a Brown Coconut

Poke at the three "eyes" on one end of your coconut shell with a clean screwdriver. One of them should give with a little pressure, allowing you to widen a hole by twisting the screwdriver around a few times. Tip the widened hole over a drinking glass and relax for a few minutes while the water drips out. Then, take the nut somewhere you can strike it with a hammer or rock until it breaks. If the meat is sticking to the shell like it usually does, break it into fairly small pieces so you can pry the meat out safely with a dull knife or edge of a spoon. I use a lot of coconuts because now I love them and this is how I do it. If you have a better way, please let me know.

• Dates

This is another luxury item that I never used much until I went raw. One reason was the inferior quality of the dried up Deglet noors that appear in stores before Christmas, in time for holiday baking, and then mercifully disappear afterwards. Deglet noor is the most common variety because it ships and stores well, but all the others I have found are superior in flavor and texture.

Try the soft, fragrant halawi, barhi, or honey dates and other varieties that are becoming more widely available. Pit a magnificent medjool and pack the opening with raw almond butter for a fast, heavenly candy. I had my first fresh medjools right off the tree while visiting Palestine in 2001, and it brought tears to my eyes from some distant racial memory of its sweet perfection.

Dates are the original whole food raw vegan sweetener and the only one mentioned in earlier raw recipe collections. They work great where their bulk, stickiness, flavor, and color make a contribution in sweet pie crusts, spice breads, cakes, and cookies. With the advent of raw agave nectar, gourmet raw vegans have more choices in dishes where the color and flavor might not be such a plus, such as some raw ice creams, icings, and coconut confections.

• Dulse

Raw fooders seem to use a lot of seaweeds, or sea vegetables as they are called. I know they are very, very good for me and this inlander is still trying to like them, but I would still rather take a bath in the stuff than eat it.

Dulse, a mild red laver from northern waters, sold dried and sometimes flaked, is so far the easiest sea vegetable for me to like. Tear it in pieces and sprinkle it over a salad with a strong vinegary dressing if your thyroid needs support. Experiment with other sea vegetables such as kelp, sea palm, hijiki, wakame, and fucus if you like.

• Durian

A large tree melon long appreciated by denizens of tropical climes, frozen whole durians are now available in Asian markets. Given the peculiar dirty-sock smell of the rind—which has nothing to do with the hauntingly desirable taste of its flesh—these paradoxes make a great offering to bring to a picnic or outdoor gathering. Split thawed durians along one of their fault lines with a knife, being careful of the sharp horny thorns. Scoop out the fruit which clings to the large seeds. Enjoy them plain or added to frozen desserts.

• Fig

A fig tree forces generosity, for all its abundant fruit ripens at the same time. If you live in a temperate area and have space (I grow figs in Portland, Oregon) plant one or two varieties. While you are waiting three years for your first fruits, make friends with neighbors who have mature trees and offer to help them with the harvest. Fresh ripe figs (the best way to eat them) don't need any gourmet treatment beyond being sliced open. Eat as many as you can in season. Some taste great frozen; the rest will have to be dried or given away. Some varieties dry better if you blend them up first to make a fruit leather.

• Goji

Also known as wolfberry, lycii, or lyceum fruit, this small berry, whose taste is reminiscent of a cross between a raisin and a cranberry, is native to China and Tibet. It is available dried from raw food web sites and also from Chinese herb suppliers, for it is prized as a medicine and tea. Goji berries became popular among the Western health elite when researchers identified in its juice the highest anti-oxidant value of anything yet tested. They are delicious in trail mixes, added to bars and cookies, or eaten out of hand. Be careful of your source. Exporters sometimes add red dye to mask poor quality and then warning labels about boiling the fruit before consuming it, which is not an option for a raw fooder.

• Jerusalem Artichoke

Related to artichokes only by a misnomer, this is a type of sunflower which stores its sun energy in tubers at the end of the growing season. The crunchy tubers are high in the good starch inulin, and need only be washed, sliced, and added to salads. But see the chapter "Soup and Crackers" for a way to prepare them that caused me to forget I was ever addicted to potato chips.

• Jicama

Pronouced hee-ka-mah, it is also called a yam bean or Fon Goot. It is a common root vegetable in Mexico, resembling a large, brown turnip in appearance but not taste. Peel the easily removed covering to reveal white flesh which is crispy and sweet, reminiscent of water chesnuts.

• Lemongrass

The stem end of these tropical grass clumps, sold in Asian stores, imparts a special Thai flavor to gourmet raw dishes. Slice small pieces across the grain and blend with liquid ingredients. If necessary, strain out any stray fibers. See the chapter "Raw Garden" for how to grow your own.

• Longan

See Lychee.

• Lotus Root

Lotus root, from a type of water lily, is a valuable part of Chinese medicine and cuisine. You can enjoy its interesting, sweetish crunchiness raw in salads by peeling and thinly slicing the roots to show off their lacy texture. Marinate it in lemon or lime juice to prevent oxidation.

• Lychee

Lychee, or litchi, along with related longan and rambutan, are small, tropical fruits encased in an easy-to-peel rind that are best eaten raw. Pop them open with your fingernail or a small knife and eat the sweet white pulp that surrounds the single nut. Offer them whole for dessert or as a conversation-starting garnish on a gourmet raw dinner plate.

• Mushrooms

When raw fooders talk about mushrooms, they don't mean those ordinary white buttons from the supermarket, but what the adventurous uncover in meadows and forests after a rainfall, or what the less well-informed can now find increasingly in markets.

Mushroom-farmed brown crimini, its big brother Portabello, oyster, and the healthful shiitake are now commonly available year round. In season, a lucky forager of gourmet markets will discover chanterelles, morels, matsutake, boletes, and other prizes.

Mushroom consumption is controversial in the raw world. On the plus side, they are delicious and help us replicate meaty flavors and textures of nostalgic memory. A raw garden burger with a slice of tomato and onion between two Portabello mushroom caps actually looks and feels somewhat like a hamburger on a bun. Many, like shiitake, maitaki, and reishi mushrooms have documented medicinal value. On the minus side, mushrooms are definitely fungus and are not recommended for yeast-elimination diets. Traces of cancer-causing chemicals have been identified even in those innocuous white buttons. If you fear mushrooms, do not use them. Fear is not good for the digestion.

• Nori

This is another sea vegetable most commonly available pressed into thin rectangular sheets for rolling sushi. Since it is dried, it can be kept in the cupboard for long periods to have on hand whenever you need it. Nori sheets are very light and pack well for traveling when you are bringing your own food. Nori works as a casing for rolling up raw pâtés and vegetable sushis. If you miss fish flavors, nori can console you. It is sold both raw and toasted in Asian markets and health food stores as well as online. Check the label to make sure that your nori is raw.

• Olives

I was relieved to learn that olives are a legitimate item for consumption by raw fooders; that is, if they are fresh, dried, or brined without pasteurizing or canning. Fresh olives are hard to come by unless you have your own tree, and all but the most devoted olive worshippers find them unpalatable. Olives dried without salt are edible and good to some tastes, especially the large Peruvian ones. Moroccan-type dried olives are very salty. Soaking and draining away some of the salt is recommended. Brined olives of all sizes, colors, and flavors can be wonderful. Thomas and I always graze the olive bars of upscale supermarkets when we are in them. An enormous olive craving emerged when I first went raw, which was lots of fun to satisfy.

• Papaya, green

You may already know that a ripe orange or yellow papaya is a mouthwatering treat whether fresh or dried. The firm, green-tasting flesh of immature papayas sold in Asian markets lends itself to shredding and bathing in lime-coconut-based marinades with Thai flavorings.

• Persimmon

Persimmons are a teardrop-shaped, seasonal delicacy. Hachiya persimmons and flat-bottomed Fuyus appear in the stores in the fall. Hachiyas are a ready-made pudding when they are soft-ripe. All you need is a spoon and a napkin. Fuyus taste good when they are still crunchy, dry well, and eventually ripen to a pudding texture also.

• Pine Nuts

The sweet, oily seed of a very large pine cone, pine nuts are best known for providing their unique flavor to pestos and can act like butterfat in gourmet raw cuisine. Pine nuts, being softer than most other raw seeds or nuts, easily blend into a creamy texture.

• Pomegranate

A red fruit with sweet-tart, juicy, red, edible seeds, pomegranates are now becoming more common, thanks to a major marketing campaign by California growers. The ruby seeds look great in fruit salads and as decorations for raw cakes, or the juice can be added to soups, sauces, and drinks.

• Rambutan

See Lychee.

• Tomatillo

This is a small, green-to-yellow, sweet-bitter fruit related to the tomato and featured in Mexican cuisine, especially salsas. Remove the paper husks before eating. They are as easy to grow as tomatoes and much favored by children.

• Wasabi

Wasabi is a beautiful, glossy-leafed plant in the mustard family with a smooth horseradish-y pungency in the roots and leaves. It is prized as a flavoring for sushi sauces and usually adulterated in commercial preparations due to its cost. You can grow your own, like I do, in a shaded, wet pot, or substitute horseradish for wasabi in recipes.

• Water Chestnut

Chinese water chestnuts, available in Asian markets, are actually tastier as well as healthier when eaten fresh. To use, simply peel off the brown coating with a knife. They add welcome crunch to salads and Chinese-inspired gourmet raw dishes.

• Yacon

Yacon, originally from South America, is now being grown in Oregon gardens, including my own. Like the Jerusalem artichoke, yacon makes edible tubers late in the growing season. The tubers are large, heavy, and watery-sweet. Also like Jerusalem artichokes, yacon tubers are high in inulin starch which benefits the pancreas. They are great peeled and sliced on a vegetable platter.

CHAPTER 4

CAKE FOR BREAKFAST

A dearly held birthday tradition from my childhood (which I may have initiated) was that the birthday girl could eat the leftover cake for breakfast the next morning. On my lucky day, I would gleefully immerse the dry-ish layers of Duncan Hines, glued together with my mother's own butter cream frosting, in a bowl of chocolate ice milk "soup"—one of my early culinary creations.

I have never forgotten the sweet joy of such breakfasts, especially the feeling of being able to eat as much as I wanted of just what I wanted unburdened by either conscience—our family was large and poor—or any awareness of how unhealthy it was. I celebrated my childhood in the 1950s before the ubiquitous, carcinogenic food dyes, artificial sweeteners, and indigestible trans-fats were proven guilty, and few knew that the tiny mercury-silvered sugar balls sprinkled on the cake (which I would sneak from the cupboard and chew like candy) could ever be a problem.

But today I have learned how to have my cake for breakfast—rich, lovely, mouthwatering cake—without incurring guilt or inflicting self damage. Raw cakes are not only good tasting but also good for you. The basic ingredients in raw cakes, pies, and cookies are fruits, nuts and flavorings. The variations are as endless as nature and your creativity. If you wish, it is fun to invite your child—inner or outer—to help mold and decorate the cake with you.

I call this "15 Years or Minutes Cake" because, if you have all the ingredients and equipment ready, 15 minutes is all it takes to put it together ready to serve. But this cake really begins with the planting of the fruit and nut trees and brings the vibration of all the loving care of the gardener and the world of nature fresh to your grateful palate.

In between the 15 years to grow the ingredients and the 15 minutes to assemble, of course, is all the time it takes you to prepare them. Start at least the night or morning before to give the nuts time to soak and re-dry if possible. You can also soak and re-dry nuts up to a week in advance and hold them in the refrigerator for the moment you need the cake. If you are able to shell the nuts yourself, perhaps with a friend over gentle conversation, you can begin the process of admiring and appreciating nature's gifts, thinking good thoughts about who you are preparing the food for and adding to the love which will be palpable in the final result.

15 YEARS OR MINUTES CAKE

This recipe makes two 3/4 inch layers for a 9 inch round cake, or crust for two 9 inch pies.

American		Metric
4 cups	Shelled fresh raw nuts (walnuts, almonds, pecans, filberts [hazelnuts], etc in any combination)	420g
2 cups	Raisins, figs, pitted dates or prunes in any combination, soaked briefly and rinsed if hard and dry	320g
	Sprinkle of unrefined salt	
	Vanilla, cinnamon, or other flavoring	
	Optional: sweeteners such as raw honey, agave, and/or stevia extract powder	
2 cups	Fresh sliced soft fruit for the filling (strawberries, mangos, papaya, ripe pear, banana, persimmon, etc.)	280g

Grind the nuts dry to an even powder in a food processor with an "S" blade. Pour into large mixing bowl. Process the dried fruits, optional sweetener, salt and flavoring in the food processor with an "S" blade until softened. Add a very little water if need be. Mix by hand with the ground nuts, or in the food processor if it is large enough. When dough holds together and tastes delicious, divide in half. Pat first half onto a cake plate (or spring form pan) and mold into a pleasing shape for the first layer.

Cover the layer with fruit slices and pat down gently. Mold the rest of the dough on top to fit. Ice with **Amazing Avocado Icing** (see below) and decorate with fruit and edible flowers if you wish.

AMAZING AVOCADO ICING
AND FRUIT FONDUE

Some raw food genius discovered that processing avocado this way results in an incredibly delicious creamy icing. Your friends will never guess the main ingredient.

American		Metric
	2 large, or 3 medium, ripe Hass avocados (Hass work best because they are highest in fat) peeled and seeded	
	1/2 teaspoon vanilla	
	Sprinkle unrefined salt	
1/3–1/2 cup	raw honey or agave nectar (start with less and adjust to taste)	85–120g
1/2 cup	raw carob powder	70g
	Optional:	
1/3 cup	ground raw cacao beans and	45g
1/3 cup	carob for a chocolate fudge icing	40g

Process the avocado, salt and sweetener with an "S" blade until blended. Add powdered carob and optional ground cacao beans. Process briefly until creamy and chocolaty brown. You can add one very ripe banana to stretch the amount of icing without affecting the texture, but it will affect the taste, somewhat, of the final result.

BREAKFAST ICED BISCOTTI

1 leftover raw cake, any amount

Slice cake into 1/2 inch thick pieces and dry them for a few hours until pliable or overnight until crisp. What results will taste like explosively flavorful iced biscotti.

BASIC NUT OR SEED MILK

Fresh nut milks only take a few minutes to make and are so much better and cheaper than packaged soy or other non-dairy milks. Save the precious pulp for the next recipe.

American		Metric
1–2 cups	fresh raw almonds or other nuts or seeds, soaked 4 hours to overnight, rinsed and drained	140–280g
2–4 cups	water	460-920ml
	Optional: Unrefined salt, flavoring, and/or sweetener	

Put nuts in blender and cover with water 1–2 times above the level of the nuts. Less water makes a richer milk: more water makes a skimmer milk. Blend at high speed until the nuts are chopped as fine as possible. This will take less than a minute in a high-speed blender, longer in a regular one. Pour the slurry into a clean nylon bag or several layers of cheesecloth draped over a colander with a bowl beneath to catch the milk. Gather it up and hold the bag tightly closed, gently "milk" your nut or seed cow until most of the liquid is pressed out. Add salt if you wish to make it taste more like cow's milk, or other desired flavors. Serve or refrigerate. Use within 4 days.

BREAKFAST BIKKIES

Leftover pulp from nut milk stays good for 3 days in my refrigerator. I usually find a delicious way like the one below to use it up before then. See the chapter "Soup and Crackers" for more variations of the basic flax cracker.

American		*Metric*
2 cups	flax seed (brown or golden)	280g
2 cups	water	460ml
	1 large whole lemon minus seeds, sliced with peel on	
1/2 cup	raw honey or equivalent sweetener	125g
	1 tablespoon cold pressed, unrefined coconut oil	
	1/2 teaspoon vanilla	
	Unrefined salt to taste	
1–2 cups	Pulp left over from making nut milk	100–200g

Place flax seeds in a strainer and rinse quickly. Put in food processor with an "S" blade in place and cover with water. Let sit at least 30 minutes up to overnight while it becomes a sticky mass. Add lemon slices, honey, coconut oil, vanilla, and salt. Process until lemon peel is fully blended. The flax seeds won't break up. Finish processing with the pulp. Spread on mesh sheets in a food dehydrator to biscuit thickness and dry until chewy or crisp.

BREAKFAST SMOOTHIES

Fast, simple, and filling.

American		Metric
1/2 cup	Raw almonds or other nuts, soaked overnight, drained and rinsed	70g
1 cup	Filtered water	230ml
	1 ripe banana	
	Fresh or frozen fruit of your choice	

Blend nuts and water until liquefied. Don't bother to strain unless you need the pulp or your blender doesn't blend well. Add banana and other fruit and blend until smooth. May be protein enhanced with 1 teaspoon of bee pollen and flavor enhanced with salt, vanilla, stevia, honey, and/or sweet spices.

KEFIR SMOOTHIES

Developing a relationship with kefir is a commitment but worth it if you can. Kefir is an ancient yogurt-like drink loaded with beneficial probiotics that can easily be made with nut milks. You'll need to acquire kefir grains to start your culture and learn how to care for them. Starter grains and good information are available online, especially at "Dom's Kefir In-site" (see Appendix, p. 173).

American		Metric
1–2 cups	Kefir cultured in almond milk	230–460ml
	1 ripe banana	
2 cups	Raspberries or blackberries, fresh or frozen	260g
	Optional: 1–3 teaspoons bee pollen	

Blend and drink. Vary the recipe with seasonal fruit combinations and flavors. I also like apple-cranberry cinnamon, pear-nutmeg, orange-pineapple, strawberry-blueberry. If you have any fresh currants, either red or black, adding a handful to the mix takes it to a new dimension. Always use a banana for thickness. The protein in bee pollen, added to kefir, will be more bio-available because the kefir begins digesting the protective coating around the pollen.

BREAKFAST SWEET BREADS

Use up Halloween pumpkins and your neighbor's zucchini (courgettes) for this recipe. You'll wish you had more nut pulp because these go down easy any time of the day.

American		Metric
4 cups	Chopped, peeled, raw pumpkin, or winter squash or zucchini (courgettes) with peel	440g
1/2 cup	Raw honey or agave nectar	125g
	1 teaspoon vanilla	
	2 tablespoons cold pressed, unrefined coconut oil	
	1 tablespoon cinnamon or pumpkin pie spice	
	Unrefined salt to taste	
2–3 cups	Nut pulp left over from making milk	200–300g
1 cup	Whole flax seed, ground in an electric mill or blender (Flax goes rancid quickly so should be ground fresh. Grinding will almost double the volume.)	140g
1 cup	Raisins	150g
1 cup	Chopped walnuts	140g

Process chopped squash, honey, vanilla, coconut oil, spice, and salt with an "S" blade of a food processor until it forms a slurry. Process in nut pulp and sufficient ground flax seed for the soft dough to hold together. Turn into a bowl and mix in raisins and chopped nuts. Form into a loaf shape. Cut 1/2 inch slices and carefully place on mesh sheets in a food dehydrator. Dry until chewy.

SIMPLE SWEET BREAD

Very easy to make. Start it the night before and enjoy it in the morning.

American		Metric
2 cups	Flax seed	280g
	Water to cover	
1/4 cup	raw honey, or agave nectar with stevia extract powder, to taste	65g
	1 tablespoon cold pressed, unrefined coconut oil	
1 cup	Walnuts	140g
1 cup	Raisins	150g
	Optional: 1–2 teaspoons cinnamon	

Rinse flaxseeds quickly in a strainer and pour into a food processor fitted with an "S" blade. Add water to cover, honey, and coconut oil. Process until mixed. Wait a few minutes to a few hours until water has been absorbed by seeds, and then pulse in walnuts and raisins. Spread dough on a mesh sheet and dehydrate until pliable or crisp—a few hours to overnight.

BANANA BREAD

We start eating this for breakfast and then snack on it all day.

American		Metric
	3–5 very ripe bananas	
1 1/2 cups	Freshly ground flax seed meal	200g
	1 tablespoon unrefined coconut oil	
	1 teaspoon cinnamon	
	Sprinkle of unrefined salt	
	Sweetener of choice if needed	
2 cups	Walnuts, soaked several hours to overnight, rinsed, drained and re-dried, or unsoaked	280g

Peel and purée bananas in a food processor fitted with an "S" blade. Mix in everything except the walnuts and blend thoroughly. Pulse in walnuts, leaving some chunks for texture. Spread dough about 1/2 inch thick on mesh dehydrator sheets to dry until pliable.

ST. JOHN'S BREAD

All of the ingredients are mentioned in the Bible. Eat reverently.

American		Metric
1/2 cup	Flax seeds	70g
1 cup	Sprouted wheat, rye, or barley	120g
1/4 cup	Raw carob powder	35g
	1/2 teaspoon powdered orange peel (or 1 teaspoon fresh grated)	
	1/2 teaspoon peppermint extract	
	2 tablespoons raw honey	
	1 tablespoon olive oil	
	Sprinkle unrefined salt	
1 cup	Almond pulp left over from making almond milk	100g
2 cups	Raisins	300g
2 cups	Raw nuts soaked, rinsed, drained, and re-dried, then chopped	280g

Rinse the flax seeds in a strainer and place in a food processor fitted with an "S" blade. Wait an hour and process in sprouted grain. Add carob, orange, peppermint, olive oil, salt, and honey and process until thoroughly mixed. Turn into a large bowl, and then mix in chopped nuts and raisins. Form small, flattened patty cakes and place on mesh dehydrator trays. Turn after cakes are dry on the bottom and finish drying until dry most of the way through.

GRAW-NOLA

I created this to see if I could duplicate the granola (muesli) of happy memory. It came out even better tasting and is a breakfast staple in our household. Graw-nola travels well and also makes nice clumps that work for a quick snack. It's good to add crunch to ice cream. For a morning meal that keeps you going well into the afternoon, eat it in a bowl with a kefir smoothie poured over it. Makes enough to fill a gallon (3.785l) jar.

American		Metric
3–4 cups	Raw buckwheat groats which will then need to be soaked and sprouted for 1–3 days (will double in amount)	420–560g
2–3 cups	Raw, hulled sunflower seeds which will need to be soaked and sprouted for 1 day	280–420g
2–3 cups	Raw hulled pumpkins seeds, then soak and sprout for 1 day	280–420g
	1 brown coconut, husked, shelled and cut into pieces	
	2 pears or apples chopped and seeded with skin remaining	
1 cup	Raisins, rinsed	150g
1/2–1 cup	Raw honey or agave nectar	125–250g
	3 tablespoons cold pressed, unrefined coconut oil	
	2 teaspoons vanilla	
	Unrefined salt, cinnamon, and stevia extract powder to taste	
	Optional:	
1–2 cups	Small, dried fruit, such as blueberries, goji berries, more raisins, chopped figs, or apricots	150–300g

Rinse and drain the groats and place in a very large mixing bowl. Roughly chop the drained sunflower and pumpkins seeds in a food processor with an "S" blade and add to mix. Rinse, drain, and pulse the pieces of coconut meat in the food processor until roughly grated. I like to leave some small chunks. Add to the bowl with other ingredients. Combine chopped pears or apples, raisins, honey, coconut oil, and any flavoring in the food processor and blend to a slurry. Fold into the other ingredients in the mixing bowl and stir until everything is well coated. Add optional dried fruit to the folding if desired. Spread mixture 1/2–3/4 inch thick on mesh sheets in the dehydrator. Dry on moderate, rotating the trays after a few hours. Finish drying on lower heat, cool, and then store in covered containers. Enjoy "as is" or with nut milk and berries. Stays fresh for several weeks, but usually doesn't stay around that long!

SIMPLE BREAKFAST CEREAL

No time to make *graw-nola*? Try this. Visiting children often ask for it at my house.

American		*Metric*
1–2 cups	Raw oat groats, soaked overnight and drained	140–280g

Raw oat groats will be soft and chewy enough to eat the next morning if you remember to put them out to soak before you go to bed. Any extra can be kept in the refrigerator for a few days. Enjoy with almond milk and fresh fruit.

BREAKFAST FRUIT MUESLI

An attainable luxury when you're traveling as well as at home.

American		*Metric*
	1–2 apples or pears, chopped small	
1 cup	Diced dates, figs or pitted prunes in any combination	150g
1/2 cup	Raisins	75g
1/2 cup	Raw hulled, sunflower seeds, soaked or unsoaked	75g
	Cinnamon to taste	
	Optional: soaked, chopped, raw almonds	

Mix it all together gratefully.

CHAPTER 5

GREEN FOOD

(SALADS, DRESSINGS, DIPS, AND SAUCES)

Most people imagine that a raw food lifestyle means salads, and nothing but salads, or perhaps salads and fruit. In a way they are right that a pure raw food diet would be just that. But add human creativity to those raw ingredients and you have the kind of tempting and satisfying eating that a diehard cooked consumer can delight in, too.

Frankly, I have never been drawn to green salads unless they were made with vibrantly fresh ingredients and a tasty dressing. My sweet tooth has me leaning towards fruits, but the rest of my body tells me I need the balancing chlorophyll just as much. Yours probably does, too.

The solution for me was to become an explorer and discoverer of salad dressings that I could easily love and easily make. As a reward for my effort, I discovered that dressings also work great as dips and sauces (and vice versa) for more elaborate raw dishes.

MAKE YOUR OWN MESCLUN SALAD
WITH BASIL HONEY MUSTARD DRESSING

Select, wash, and cut or tear into bite size pieces any combination of the freshest and best greens available. Choose from gourmet lettuces, mustards, mache, endive, arugula (rocket), radicchio, cabbage, kale, collard, chard, sunflower sprouts, micro greens, dandelion, and edible weeds. Serve tossed or drizzled with this sweet-tangy basil-drenched dressing. Every single person, raw or cooked, to whom I have offered this loves it. Plan ahead to have fresh basil year round by blending fresh basil in season with olive oil, freezing the mix in ice cube trays and storing in zip lock bags in your freezer. For this recipe, use 2 or 3 frozen basil cubes and less oil.

American		Metric
	1 large bunch chopped, fresh basil—the more you can fill up your blender the better	
1 cup	Extra virgin olive oil	230ml
1/2 cup	Raw apple cider vinegar	115ml
1/4–1/3 cup	Raw honey or agave nectar	60–90g
	1–2 teaspoons yellow mustard powder	
	1–2 teaspoons unrefined salt to taste	

Put it all together in the blender and liquefy. It keeps in the refrigerator for at least a week.

HONEY MUSTARD DRESSING

Same as above but omit the basil. Almost as good.

FRENCH TARRAGON DRESSING

Dry tarragon in the summer when your plant grows exuberantly and use it year round for this.

American		Metric
1/2 cup	Raw apple cider vinegar	115ml
1 cup	Extra virgin olive oil	230ml
	2 Roma tomatoes, chopped	
	1–2 tablespoons dried tarragon	
	Unrefined salt and pepper to taste	

Optional: to make a protein-packed, creamy dressing, blend in several tablespoons of soaked and drained pumpkin or sunflower seeds. Experiment with different herbs.

Put everything in a blender and liquefy.

RASPBERRY VINAIGRETTE

Very simple, very delicious.

American		Metric
1/2 cup	Raw apple cider vinegar	115ml
1 cup	Extra virgin olive oil	230ml
1 cup	Fresh raspberries	130g
1/3 cup	Raw honey or agave or to taste	90g
	Unrefined salt to taste	

Put everything in a blender and liquefy.

THAI DRESSING

Good over shredded cabbage, strong flavored greens, and chopped vegetables. No need to waste the flavor and nutrition of the jalapeño seeds, which will break up in the blender.

American		Metric
	2–3 limes, juiced	
	2 tablespoons coconut oil	
	1 jalapeño pepper chopped, with seeds	
	2 inch piece of lemon grass, chopped	
	1 bunch fresh mint, chopped	
1/3–1/2 cup	Raisins	50–75g
	Unrefined salt to taste	
	Water if needed to blend	

Put lime juice, coconut oil, and jalapeño in blender and liquefy. Pulse in rest of the ingredients and finish blending.

WASABI SAUCE OR DIP

Wasabi leaves provide the pretty pale green color. Throw in a little kale, or spinach if you are using horseradish, for the same effect. This is a mild version. For a stronger flavor, add more horseradish or mustard.

American		Metric
1/2 cup	Raw apple cider vinegar	115ml
	1 lemon, juiced	
1/2 cup	Extra virgin olive oil	115ml
1 cup	Raw hulled sunflower seeds, soaked at least a few hours to overnight, drained	140g
	1 whole wasabi plant, leaves and root, washed and chopped, or substitute a 2 inch piece of fresh chopped horseradish root	
	1/2 teaspoon yellow mustard powder	
	Unrefined salt to taste	

Put everything in a blender or food processor and blend until smooth.

SWEET FENNEL SEED DRESSING

An interesting fruit dip or dressing for fruit salads.

American		Metric
	Juice of 1 large lemon	
	1 stalk of celery, chopped	
	2 tablespoons raw honey or agave nectar	
1/2 cup	Raw almonds, soaked and drained	70g
	1 tablespoon fennel seeds	
	Water to blend	
	Dash unrefined salt to taste	

Place celery, lemon juice, and honey in blender and liquefy. Add almonds and fennel seeds and blend until smooth, adding water in small amounts if necessary. Salt to taste.

SUNNY SESAME DRESSING

American		Metric
	Juice of 2 oranges	
1/4 cup	Extra virgin olive oil	65ml
	3 tablespoons unhulled sesame seeds, soaked a few hours and drained	
	1 tablespoon unpasteurized miso, any flavor	
	2 tablespoons fresh ginger	

Put everything in a blender and blend until smooth.

FRESH AND RAW SALSA

These are the basic ingredients. Adjust to suit your palate.

American		Metric
	3 medium vine ripe tomatoes, sliced	
	1 small red onion	
	1–2 jalapeño peppers with seeds	
1/3 cup	Raw apple cider vinegar	75ml
	2 cloves garlic	
	Unrefined salt to taste	
1/3–1/2 cup	Dried tomatoes cut small	40–60g
	Optional: pulse in 1 bunch fresh, chopped cilantro (coriander leaf)	

Pulse everything, except the dried tomatoes, in a food processor with an "S" blade. Stir in dried tomatoes. Allow to soften for an hour or so and pulse together with the rest. If you are in a hurry and don't mind a more puréed texture, pulse everything a blender instead.

TOMATILLO SAUCE

My friend, Laurie Wheeler, who shares this recipe, says her two children devour this sauce plain. Make extra to freeze for later.

American		*Metric*
	7–8 medium tomatillos, washed, with paper husks removed.	
1/4 cup	Chopped celery	25g
1/4 cup	Sweet onion, chopped	25g
	1 tablespoon lemon juice	
	Unrefined salt to taste	
	Optional for grown-ups: 1 mild to hot chili pepper	

Pulse ingredients in a food processor with an "S" blade until chopped and blended.

CORIANDER RAITA

Serve this to cool off raw curries or as a dip.

American		*Metric*
	1 whole cucumber, diced small	
1/2 cup	Pine nuts	70g
	1 lemon, juiced	
	1 lime, juiced	
	1 bunch cilantro (coriander), leaves only	
	1 bunch mint, leaves only	
	1 teaspoon chili powder	
	Unrefined salt to taste	

Place diced cucumber in bowl. Liquefy pine nuts with lemon and lime juice in blender. Briefly blend in the remaining ingredients. Stir into bowl with cucumber.

RAINBOW SALAD
WITH CREAMY DRESSING

This recipe is courtesy of my friend, Rosi Goldsmith, www.devacommunion.org, who leads workshops on communicating and cooperating with the nature kingdom and who works intuitively with plants to create recipes. Beautiful, hearty, tasty, and filling, this meets the protein requirements of those with a high need.

American		*Metric*
	Vegetables	
	Any of the following in any combination:	
	Red cabbage • Cauliflower • Red or yellow peppers • Carrots • Leafy greens	
	Dressing	
	Juice of 1 large or 2 medium lemons	
1/4 cup	Olive oil	60ml
1/2–1 cup	Water to desired thickness	115–230ml
2 cups	Raw, hulled sunflower seeds and hazelnuts in any combination, soaked, and sprouted	280g
2 cups	Mung beans or lentils which have been sprouted 3 days and are at their sweetest	260g
	3 tablespoons fresh thyme	
	1 1/2 tablespoons fresh sage	
	1 1/2 tablespoons dried Italian herbs	
	Unrefined salt to taste	

Wash, chop, and toss vegetables together in a large salad bowl. Set aside. Place the dressing ingredients in blender and blend until smooth. Serve over chopped vegetables or as a vegetable dip.

JIM'S SIGNATURE SALAD

We were always glad to see Jim at our weekly potlucks because we could count on him to bring some version of this. At home, he makes this his main meal by adding soaked sunflower or pumpkin seeds for crunch and protein.

American		Metric
	Shredded cabbage, kale, chard, or collard greens in any combination, enough to fill a large bowl	
	1 large onion, thinly sliced	
	1 red pepper, sliced	
	Optional: 2–3 chopped tomatoes, chopped celery	
1/2 cup	Nama Shoyu unpasteurized soy sauce	115ml
	Juice of 2–3 limes or lemons (or substitute apple cider vinegar)	
	2–3 cloves garlic, minced	
1 cup	Extra virgin olive oil	230ml

Mix soy sauce, lime juice, garlic, and olive oil together and stir into salad ingredients.

FIRST FRUITS SALAD

Two things that overwinter in my garden and ripen early together are fava (broad) beans and artichokes. Formerly, I loved them cooked, and now I love them raw with this simple Italian treatment. Use the best tasting olive oil you can find. When the vegetables are all gone, add some chopped greens to the left over marinade and enjoy an easy, second-generation salad.

American		Metric
	Juice of 2 lemons	
1/2 cup	Extra virgin olive oil	115ml
	2–3 crushed garlic cloves	
	Unrefined salt to taste	
2 cups	Freshly shelled fava (broad) beans	200g
	Hearts of 2–4 raw artichokes with tough leaves and choke removed, sliced thin	

Mix the marinade ingredients and pour over shelled fava (broad) beans first. Stir artichoke slices into marinade as they are prepared to prevent browning from oxidation. Cover and try to wait at least a little while for the vegetables to absorb some marinade. This is a good make-ahead dish which improves in the refrigerator over the course of a day or two.

HOLY LAND BREAKFAST SALAD

On a trip to Israel and Palestine even before we were raw, we enjoyed some combination of tomatoes and cucumbers with every breakfast. For a complete meal, serve with **Kefir Labne** (see p. 96), **Hummus** (see p. 111) and **Zaatar Crisps** (see p. 86).

American		Metric
1/4 cup	Raw apple cider vinegar or lemon juice	70ml
1/4 cup	Extra virgin olive oil	70ml
	Unrefined salt to taste	
	6 vine ripe tomatoes, sliced	
	2 cucumbers, sliced	
	1 onion chopped fine	
	Optional: Dash of balsamic vinegar	

Stir vegetables gently together with the other ingredients.

PRETTY YAM SALAD

Another contribution from Rosi and the devas.

American   *Metric*

Salad

1 large yam or sweet potato, peeled and
sliced into thin matchsticks or grated

6 stalks celery, sliced thin

1 beet, grated

Leafy greens or kale, tough stems removed, and chopped

1/2 cup	Raw, hulled pumpkin seeds, soaked a few hours to overnight, rinsed, drained, and re-dried	70g

Creamy Dressing

1/2 cup	Raw, hulled sunflower seeds, soaked a few hours to overnight, rinsed and drained	70g
1/2 cup	Extra virgin olive oil	115ml
1/2 cup	Raw apple cider vinegar and juice of 1 orange or juice of 2 lemons and oranges	115ml

2 tablespoons dried dill weed or 2 tablespoons Italian herbs

Other fresh herbs, as desired, such as thyme,
mint, rosemary, and celery seed

1 apple, chopped

Unrefined salt to taste

Combine dressing ingredients in blender and blend until smooth, adding water to thin if desired. Marinate yam, celery and beet in dressing for one hour. Serve over chopped greens sprinkled with pumpkin seeds.

TWO BEAN SALAD

This is both crunchier than I remember in its cooked incarnation and lacking in kidney beans, but I still like it.

American		Metric
2 cups	Fresh, tender string beans, de-stemmed and cut small	200g
1 cup	Dried garbanzo beans (chick peas), soaked over night, rinsed, and sprouted for 1–2 days (will double in amount)	140g
	1 cucumber, diced	
	1 sweet onion, diced	
	2 cloves garlic, crushed	
1/2 cup	Extra virgin olive oil	115ml
1/4 cup	Raw apple cider vinegar	60ml
	Juice of 1 lemon	
	1/2–1 teaspoon unrefined salt, to taste	
	Optional: Small pieces of sea vegetables	

Marinate beans with the other ingredients in a serving bowl for several hours or in the refrigerator.

Cole Slaw

Makes a lot to feed a crowd or will welcome you home to your refrigerator for several days.

American		Metric
1 cup	Raw apple cider vinegar	230ml
1/2 cup	Extra virgin olive oil	115ml
1/2 cup	Raw honey or agave nectar	125g
	1 teaspoon of unrefined salt or to taste	
	1 head green cabbage	
	6 medium carrots, chopped	
	Optional:	
1/2 cup	For a creamy dressing, add soaked sprouted seeds or nuts	70g

Grate cabbage in batches to fit your food processor fitted with an "S" blade and place in large bowl. Do the same with carrots and mix together with grated cabbage. Blend or stir wet ingredients and mix in.

Bossanova Salad

This salad, named for the aforementioned nightclub in Portland, Oregon, consoled us on a recent US election eve at a "Rock the Vote" party where it was featured on a buffet table decorated with little paper flags.

American		Metric
	Juice of 1 orange	
	Juice of 1 lemon	
4 cups	Grated carrots	400g
1 cup	Dried cherries	100g

Mix together and serve in a glass bowl with or without paper flags.

YOUNG SALAD

Young green coconuts and papayas grow up fast in this pungent Thai environment.

American		Metric
	Juice of 2 limes	
	2 tablespoons lemongrass, chopped	
	1 tablespoon ginger root, chopped	
1/2 cup	Water from a green coconut	115ml
	1 jalapeño or Thai chili pepper	
	1 tablespoon unrefined coconut oil	
	2 tablespoons raw honey or agave nectar	
	1/2 teaspoon unrefined salt or to taste	
	1 bunch cilantro (coriander leaf)	
	1 bunch mint	
	1 small green papaya	
	Meat of 1 "green" coconut, sliced into thin ribbons	
	Variation: Use thinly sliced, peeled lotus root with, or instead of, green papaya	

Prepare dressing first by liquefying lime juice, coconut water, jalapeño , lemongrass, ginger, honey, coconut oil, and salt in a blender or food processor. Pulse in mint and cilantro (coriander leaf), leaving some small bits of leaf if desired. Peel and thinly shred green papaya with the julienne blade of a mandoline or in a food processor or a vegetable spiralizer. (A spiralizer is a fun but fussy gadget that turns firm vegetables and fruits into angel hair pasta. One popular brand is called Saladacco.) Mix with julienned coconut meat and dressing.

FRUIT CHAT MASALA

Surprise your friends with these sophisticated flavors at a potluck. Use seasonal fruits.

Juice of 1 lemon

1 tablespoon ginger, minced fine

1 jalapeño pepper, seeded and minced fine

1 small bunch mint, minced

1 tablespoon fennel seeds

Unrefined salt

Summer version

American		*Metric*
	1 small honeydew or other melon, peeled and cut into attractive, bite-size pieces	
2 cups	Sliced strawberries and/or grapes or figs, in any combination	260g
	1 firm-ripe papaya, peeled, seeded, and sliced or substitute other summer fruit	

Fall version

5 crisp organic apples, seeded and sliced with peel

2–4 Asian pears or Western pears, seeded and sliced

2 kiwis, sliced

Optional: Pomegranate seeds and tangerine slices to garnish

Prepare summer or winter fruits and arrange in serving bowl or platter. Sprinkle with lemon juice to coat. Mix spices and remaining ingredients together and toss over fruit.

WALDORF SALAD
WITH ALMOND MAYONNAISE

American		*Metric*
	Almond Mayonnaise	
	Juice of 1 large lemon or 2 small lemons	
1/2 cup	Extra virgin olive oil	115ml
1/2 cup	Soaked raw almonds, drained	70g
	1/2 teaspoon yellow mustard powder	
	2–3 teaspoons raw honey or agave nectar	
	1/2–1 teaspoon unrefined salt or to taste	
	Salad	
	3–4 crisp organic apples, seeded and roughly diced	
2 cups	Seedless grapes, halved if you wish	260g
1 cup	Chopped celery	120g
1 cup	Chopped, raw walnuts, soaked a few hours to overnight, rinsed, drained and re-dried, or unsoaked	140g

Place lemon juice, honey, salt, mustard powder and olive oil in blender with 1/4 cup (35g) of the almonds. Blend until smooth, adding more almonds for thickness and water if necessary to blend. Just before serving, mix mayonnaise with apples, grapes, celery, and chopped walnuts in a large bowl.

DRINK YOUR GREENS

Don't like kale? Don't chew well if you do? Try this minty green lemonade and you won't need to chew or even taste your greens to benefit from their abundant available calcium and other phytonutrients.

American		*Metric*
	1 bunch kale with stems, washed and chopped	
	1 large bunch mint with stems, chopped	
	Juice of 4 large lemons or 6 limes	
1/2 cup	Raw honey or agave nectar	115g
	Dash unrefined salt	
	Water	

Put everything in a blender and fill the rest of the way with water. Amount of sweetener can be adjusted by replacing some of the honey or agave with stevia extract, or with some fresh stems from your own plant. Blend to a coarse slurry. Strain juice through a nut milk bag or several layers of cheesecloth by squeezing over a pouring bowl or pitcher.

EMERALD SMOOTHIE

My fruit-loving husband created this when I told him he should eat more greens. It's a beautiful green color and tastes of fruit, not spinach.

1 ripe pear, washed, pitted and chopped
2 oranges, peeled and chopped
1 bunch spinach, washed and chopped
water to desired thickness

Combine everything in a blender until smooth.

CRUNCHIES

I came up with this recipe to replace the popcorn we used to love with cheese, butter, and soy sauce. Keep these on hand to top salads or snack on all by themselves.

American		Metric
2 cups	Raw, hulled sunflower seeds, soaked overnight and drained	280g
1/4 cup	Nama Shoyu or other unpasteurized soy sauce	60ml
	2 tablespoons nutritional yeast powder or flakes	
	1 teaspoon unrefined salt	
	1/4 teaspoon cayenne powder or more if you like it hot	

Stir everything together and dry on solid sheets of your dehydrator overnight or until crunchy.

SEAWEED CRUNCHY CROUTONS

One more way I've found to enjoy what's good for me!

American		Metric
2 cups	Raw, hulled sunflower seeds, soaked overnight and drained	280g
1/4 cup	Powdered sea vegetables	35g
	2 teaspoons unrefined salt or to taste	

To powder sea vegetables, take whatever dried seaweed you have or buy some dulse and pulverize in a dry blender. Stir the powder and salt into the wet sunflower seeds and dry gently on dehydrator sheets for a few hours until crisp.

DISAPPEARING KALE

Now you see it, now you don't. This recipe literally disappears off the dehydrating trays, it is so good. People who would never think of eating kale crave this.

American		Metric
	1 large bunch of kale	
1/4 cup	Nama Shoyu soy sauce	60ml
1/4 cup	Extra virgin olive oil	60ml
	1 tablespoon raw apple cider vinegar	
	Optional: 1 head of broccoli, chopped	

Wash kale, remove toughest stem ends, and chop roughly. Mix liquid ingredients and stir in to coat kale and optional broccoli. Spread on mesh dehydrator trays and dry gently for an hour or so until warm but not crisp.

CHAPTER 6

SOUPS AND CRACKERS

Raw soup outshines the boiled-to-death version in quality, taste, and ease of preparation. If you have a blender, you can make a delicious soup for one or many in minutes. Blending releases the bold flavors of fresh herbs more than you might be used to. Balance them as needed with judicious amounts of sweetener, salt, oil, or sour ingredients in recipes. In the winter, raw soups can be served comfortably warm to the touch without killing enzymes. The last remaining use I have for my oven is to heat soup bowls or plates before adding the food to preserve the warmth. Raw soups should be made as close to serving time as possible because after a few hours the enzymes which have been released by breaking down the cellular structures in the blender begin to digest your soup and change the flavor. Leftover raw soups can be resurrected as a base for pâtés or as a flavorful liquid ingredient in crackers.

AVOCADO ISLAND CONSOMMÉ

My husband, Thomas, created this classy light start to a 5 course gourmet raw feast or simple supper.

American		Metric
	1 bunch celery, juiced. Makes about 2 cups.	
	1–2 limes, juiced	
1/4 cup	Extra virgin olive oil	60ml
	Unrefined salt and pepper to taste	
	1 ripe avocado, cut into chunks	
	Optional: 1 shallot, minced	

Combine juices and shallot, if desired, in blender and blend until smooth. Pour consommé over avocado chunks and serve.

TOMATO BISQUE

This delicious soup evolved from simply blending soaked almonds into a fresh marinara sauce.

American		Metric
4 cups	Chopped, vine ripe tomatoes	520g
1/2 cup	Extra virgin olive oil	115ml
	2 chopped shallots	
	2 cloves garlic	
1/2–1 cup	Chopped fresh basil	25–50g
	1 tablespoon chopped fresh oregano	
	1 sprig fresh rosemary, stem removed	
	1/4–1/2 teaspoon cinnamon	
1 cup	Dried tomatoes	150g
1 cup	Raw almonds, soaked and drained	140g
	Unrefined salt and pepper to taste	
	Fresh rosemary or parsley for garnish	

Place tomatoes, shallots, garlic, olive oil, herbs, and cinnamon in blender and blend until smooth. Add dried tomatoes and soften for an hour or so. Blend. Add soaked almonds and blend again. Taste for seasonings and garnish.

BORSCHT

This recipe is an adaptation of one developed by the Boutenko raw family and shared with thousands of their students and guests over the years. See their web site at www.rawfamily.com

American		*Metric*
	Juice of 4 oranges	
	Juice of 2 lemons	
1/2 cup	Extra virgin olive oil	115ml
1 cup	Water	230ml
	4 beets, chopped	
	4 fresh or dried bay leaves	
	1/2–1 teaspoon unrefined salt	
	1 small cabbage, shredded	
	1–2 avocados, cut in chunks	

Put everything except cabbage and avocado in blender and purée well. Pour into large serving bowl over cabbage and avocado chunks.

COOL FENNEL SOUP

American		*Metric*
	1 bulb fennel with greens, chopped	
	Juice of 3 lemons	
1/2 cup	Extra virgin olive oil	115ml
1 cup	Celery, chopped	100g
	1/2–1 teaspoon unrefined salt	
	Sweeten to taste—a small amount of stevia extract powder works well	

Put everything in a blender and purée. Taste and adjust seasoning if needed.

HALLOWEEN SOUP

This savory soup feeds a crowd. Serve inside a hollowed out pumpkin for fun.

American		Metric
2 cups	Carrots, chopped	200g
1 cup	Water	230ml
1/2 cup	Extra virgin olive oil	115ml
	4 stalks celery, chopped	
	1 large onion, chopped	
	3 cloves garlic	
ab.4 cups	1 pumpkin or winter squash, peeled and chopped	ab.400g
	1 tablespoon fresh sage, minced	
	1 tablespoon fresh thyme, minced	
	1 tablespoon fresh rosemary, minced	
	Unrefined salt and pepper to taste	
1 cup	Kalamata or other black olives, pitted and chopped	120g

Purée carrots, onion, celery, and garlic with water and olive oil in blender. Add chopped squash a little at a time and purée. Pulse in herbs and seasonings. Pour into serving pumpkin and stir in olives.

POM POME SOUP

Serve this in the fall when pears and pomegranates are in season. It's a beautiful pink color and easy to make.

4 pomegranates, juiced
4 soft, ripe pears, seeded and chopped
Nutmeg powder

Cut pomegranates in half and juice with a citrus juicer. Strain if necessary. Combine in blender with pears. Serve cold with a sprinkle of nutmeg.

CUCURBIT CURRY SOUP

American		Metric
4 cups	Winter squash or pumpkin, chopped	400g
	Juice of 4 oranges	
	2 cloves garlic	
	1 tablespoon or more curry powder, to taste	
	3 tablespoons fresh ginger, chopped	
1/2 cup	Extra virgin olive oil	115ml
	Unrefined salt to taste	

Blend everything together until smooth.

GAZPACHO BLANCO

Even the non-raw enjoy the familiar red version redolent of tomatoes in high summer. You might like this even better, and you can make it when tomatoes are out of season.

American		Metric
1 lb	Seedless green grapes	450g
2 cups	Thick almond milk	460ml
	Juice of 1 lemon	
	2 cucumbers, chopped	
	1 shallot	
	1 clove garlic	
	Unrefined salt and pepper to taste	

To make thick almond milk, soak 2 cups (280g) raw almonds several hours to overnight, drain and put in blender with 2 cups (460ml) water. Blend and strain through a nylon mesh bag or several layers of cheese-cloth. Refrigerate pulp for another use. Wash grapes well, reserve a few, and place the rest in blender with the other ingredients. Purée. Serve chilled with halved grapes for garnish.

MAIZE MEDLEY SOUP

American		Metric
	4 fresh ears of corn, cut off the cob	
	4–6 vine ripe tomatoes	
	1 cucumber, chopped	
	1 jalapeño , chopped, with seeds	
	1 shallot or small onion	
	1 clove garlic	
1/2 cup	Extra virgin olive oil	115ml
	1 bunch mixed fresh herbs, such as basil, parsley, cilantro (coriander leaf), oregano, rosemary	
	Unrefined salt and pepper to taste	

Wait until assembling soup to cut corn off the cob. Place everything, except corn and herbs, in a food processor fitted with an "S" blade and purée. Pulse in corn and herbs.

SANGRIA SUMMER SOUP
WITH FROZEN NUT CREAM

American		Metric
4 cups	Ripe plums, pitted	520g
2 cups	Fresh raspberries, redcurrants, or blackberries in any combination	260g
	1 orange, juiced	
	1 lemon, juiced	
	Unrefined salt and sweetener to taste	

Macadamia Nut Ice Cream or any frozen nut cream (see p. 153)

Liquefy plums and berries with orange and lemon juices in blender. Add salt and sweetener to taste. Before serving, stir in large chunks of frozen nut cream.

SOUP TO GO

To have this ready when you want it, dry vegetables in season and store in tightly capped, glass jars. This soup powder can also be used to quickly enrich the taste of any other savory dish.

Dried leeks • Dried onions • Dried mushrooms • Dried tomatoes • Dried parsley • Dried carrots • Dried red peppers • Dried sweet potatoes • Dried squash • Dried greens, especially kale and spinach

Unrefined salt

1 tablespoon dried herbs, such as thyme, sage, oregano, basil, rosemary, garlic, cumin

Optional: Fresh sprouts, such as sunflower, mung bean, clover, or the like

Place 1–2 cups (120–240g) dried vegetables from above list in any combination with salt and herbs in a dry blender. Blend to a fine powder. Store in an air-tight bag or tightly closed jar for traveling. Reconstitute in somewhat hot water or almond milk. Drink warm. Stir in fresh sprouts for a filling raw stew.

RAW FOOD CHAIN CRACKERS

Keep your dehydrator humming and your cracker jars filled by giving leftover soups and pâtés another chance at life.

American		Metric
2 cups	Any leftover raw soup or pâté	230ml
2 cups	Flax seed	280g
	Unrefined salt to taste	

Briefly rinse flax seed in a strainer. Combine in a food processor fitted with an "S" blade, or a blender. Pulse to mix. Let sit until liquid is absorbed, and then finish processing. Spread dough on mesh sheets and dry until crisp.

GIVE US THIS DAY
OUR DAILY BREAD CRACKERS

These are our house crackers, and most people find the taste very good and comforting. They are quick to make when you have the almond pulp available and great to have around at all times when the urge to snack strikes.

American		Metric
2 cups	Flax seeds	280g
	Water	
	1 tablespoon extra virgin olive oil	
	2 tablespoons nutritional yeast	
	1–2 teaspoons unrefined salt	
1–2 cups	Almond pulp left over from making milk	230–460ml
	Delicious variation: Add	
1/2–1 cup	Soaked and drained, unhulled brown sesame seeds to the mix	70–140g

Briefly rinse the flax seeds in a strainer. Place in a food processor fitted with an "S" blade and cover with water. Let sit until congealed into a mass, about hour up to overnight. Add remaining ingredients and process until mixed. Spread the dough on mesh dehydrator sheets to desired thickness and dry until crisp.

ZAATAR CRISPS

Zaatar is a Middle Eastern spice blend with thyme, sumac, and sesame that can be found in specialty stores. If you make your own from foraged sumac, use the common red berries, not the poisonous white ones!

American		Metric
2 cups	Flax seed	280g
	Water	
	2 tablespoons extra virgin olive oil	
	1–2 teaspoons unrefined salt, or to taste	
1/2 cup	Pulp left over from making almond or other nut milk	115ml
1 cup	Unhulled brown sesame seeds, soaked a few hours, rinsed and drained.	140g
	2 tablespoons prepared zaatar blend or	
	1 tablespoon powdered thyme and 1 tablespoon powdered sumac	

Rinse flax seeds briefly in a strainer. Place in a food processor fitted with an "S" blade and cover with water. Let sit until congealed into a mass, half an hour to overnight. Process in remaining ingredients, except zaatar, and spread on mesh dehydrator sheets. Generously sprinkle with zaatar and dry until crisp.

GARZUKES

You will be begging for your neighbor's zucchini (courgettes) after you try these.

American		Metric
	3 small to medium zucchini (courgettes), any type	
1/2 cup	Extra virgin olive oil	115ml
	4 cloves garlic	
	2 teaspoons unrefined salt	

Blend olive oil, garlic, and salt in a blender, food processor, or mortar. Cut zucchini (courgettes) in half crosswise and slice very thin lengthwise. A mandoline or v-slicer can do this perfectly in a few minutes. Brush slices lightly with oil mixture—one side is sufficient—and spread on mesh dehydrator sheets to dry until pliable or crisp as desired.

CHAPATTI BREAD

A great high protein, low-carb recipe from raw chef John Larsen to scoop up a soup, sauce, **Vishnu's Pâté** (see p. 128) or enjoy alone as a snack (order-rawfood@vegemail.com).

American		Metric
3 cups	Sprouted chickpeas *	
3 cups	Almond flour **	
1/4 cup	Flax seed, ground	35g
	Unprocessed salt to taste	
	2 tablespoons nutritional yeast	
1 cup	Water	230ml
	2 tablespoons cold pressed grape seed oil	

In food processor combine the sprouted chickpeas and oil. Process for 2 minutes, scraping the sides of bowl several times to ensure an even consistency. Empty this purée into a large mixing bowl and add all remaining ingredients except the water. Mix with your hands, adding water slowly. After it is thoroughly mixed allow it to set for 5 minutes. Roll the dough into balls approximately the size of a golf ball. Place the ball between two non-stick dehydrator sheets, using a rolling pin flatten into a circular patty roughly 1/2 inch thick. Remove top dehydrator sheet and transfer bread onto another non-stick dehydrator sheet. Repeat for remaining dough, placing 6 breads per sheet. Dehydrate at 105 degrees for 3 hours. Turn over, removing the non-stick dehydrator sheet and continue dehydrating for another 4 hours.

*** For Sprouted Chickpeas.** Begin by thoroughly rinsing your chickpeas. Place in a large bowl adding enough water to cover all the chickpeas and allow to soak for 12 hours. Pour off soak water and rinse off in a colander. Transfer back to bowl and allow to sprout for 3 days, rinsing twice a day.

**** For Almond Flour.** Make 2 batches of almond milk using 3 cups (420g) of almonds per batch, to approximately 5 cups (1.15l) of water. Using a wire mesh strainer, strain the almond milk, pushing the pulp with a spoon to extract as much moisture as possible. Spread the pulp onto a non-stick dehydrator sheet and dehydrate at 105 degrees for 8 hours. Grind the dry pulp in a Vita-Mix or other high powered blender until you achieve a flour consistency.

CURRIED FLAX CRACKERS

My friend, Rosi, and her friends in the deva kingdom came up with this recipe for us.

American		Metric
1 cup	Sprouted buckwheat	120g
3 cups	Golden flax, soaked overnight	420g
	1 1/2 inches fresh turmeric root or 1 teaspoon powder	
	1 teaspoon dried curry powder	
	1 teaspoon coriander powder	
	1 teaspoon cumin, ground	
1 cup	Soaked hazelnuts, ground separately and processed with the rest of the ingredients	140g
	Unrefined salt to taste	

Spread inch thick on mesh trays and dry until crisp.

Variation: Divide batter in half, add cup water to one half, spread inch thick. Dry until crisp. Will form pocket in the middle.

HALLOWEEN PUMPKIN SEEDS

Drying the seeds in a dehydrator renders them as crisp as in the oven without burning or killing the nutrients.

Seeds scooped from a fresh pumpkin or squash, any amount
Unrefined salt

Separate seeds and place on solid dehydrator trays. Don't bother to wash off pulp. Sprinkle with salt. Dry until crisp.

CHILI PISTACHIOS

Raw food is not supposed to be addictive, but these can be. Chad Sarno (www.rawchef.org) created this recipe and shares it willingly with us.

American		Metric
2 cups	Pistachios (almonds work as well), soaked a few hours and drained	280g
	2 tablespoons chili powder	
	1 tablespoon onion powder	
	1 tablespoon unrefined salt	
	Optional: 1 tablespoon cumin powder	

Stir seasonings to coat wet nuts. Spread on a solid dehydrator sheet and dry until crisp.

SUNCHOKE CHIPS

I used to think I had way too many Jerusalem artichoke plants around the garden because they sprout from every tiny bit of tuber accidentally left in the ground. After discovering this treatment, I don't think that anymore, but eagerly await the first harvest in October and carefully steward my stash well into spring if I can.

Fresh Jerusalem artichoke tubers, the more the better

Extra virgin olive oil

Unrefined salt

Variation: try this with other firm vegetables such
as sweet potatoes, turnips, kohlrabi, and rutabagas (swedes).

Carefully wash but do not peel tubers. Slice thinly—a mandoline works best and quickest. Place in a bowl and add a small amount of olive oil, gently stirring to coat. Place 1/4 inch thick on mesh dehydrator sheets and sprinkle with salt. Dry until crisp and store in covered jars.

CHAPTER 7

CHEESE DREAMS

In order to go raw and successfully stay raw in a cooked world after a lifetime of cooked eating habits, memories, and expectations, most of us will need to address our food cravings, not ignore or suppress them. In our Body Electronics healing work, we have a saying, "What you resist, persists." Resisting eating old foods that tempt you will be a constant struggle, so surrender to some tempting new foods instead. When I embraced living food, I searched raw recipe books for what looked most satisfying and indulged in that until my cravings passed. With this approach, I have been a 100% raw fooder without a slip while some of my more ideologically raw friends, who disdain the bells and whistles of raw gourmet, still wrestle with temptation and sometimes lose.

The toughest transition for me was leaving behind my ingrained cheesetarian ways. I thought I might gorge on raw nut and seed cheeses instead, but that's not what happened. Smaller amounts were strangely satisfying and the effort of preparing them somehow stopped my habit of unconscious overeating. It's also true that no raw "pizza" yet revealed tastes or feels much like the cheesy offerings of the cooked world.

That said, raw copycat dishes are an entertaining and interesting way into raw cuisine for many people. After some years eating exclusively raw food, it is likely you will find yourself satisfied with more simple preparations. Taste buds refine, assimilation improves, cravings melt away. No hurry. Take the time to enjoy some of these artistic dishes while you are growing healthier and more balanced on gourmet raw and living food.

ABOUT RAW CHEESES

Like dairy cheese, most raw cheeses made with nut or seed milk are prepared or flavored with a living culture. The most common ones are miso, kefir, rejuvalac, and whatever happens to be in the air. It seems to me that clever raw cheese makers could acquire some of the classic cheese cultures like Cheddar and Roquefort and do some experimenting. I commend this to raw entrepreneurs as an area for research and product development.

Nutritional yeast, which has been heated and is no longer alive, may be used to give a cheese flavor and B vitamin boost to raw dishes. Lemon juice mimics the tang of aged cheese and helps curdle the milk. Puréed red pepper adds an orange color. Using high fat nuts like macadamia and pine nuts or adding a little olive oil increases richness and taste. Partially drying a soft cheese creates a chewier texture. Strong flavors associated with cheese dishes, such as the garlic, salt, and pine nuts in pesto can be so pronounced in raw copycat food that no one misses the cheese.

Raw cheeses may be made a few days ahead of time and refrigerated, but will not keep as long as dairy cheeses.

SIMPLE NUT OR SEED YOGURT

This is very easy. The flavor will vary with the raw ingredients. More oily nuts and seeds will make a richer yogurt. All can be mixed with fruit, fruit syrups, or raw sweeteners and flavorings.

American		Metric
2 cups	Raw almonds, walnuts, hazelnuts, sunflower, pumpkin, or sesame seeds in any combination, soaked and drained, or pine nuts and macadamia nuts unsoaked.	280g
3 cups	Water	690ml
	Optional: Open 1 acidophilus capsule and stir contents into liquid before fermenting	

Place nuts or seeds with some water in blender and blend until smooth. Add more water as needed to attain a heavy cream consistency. Strain through a nylon mesh bag or several layers of cheesecloth, reserving pulp for another use. (Pine nuts and macadamia nuts do not need to be strained.) Cover cream with a clean towel and let it sit in a warm place, such as on top of a working dehydrator, for about 8 hours until pleasantly sour. If separation occurs, decant the creamy layer and eat that.

ALMOND SOUR CREAM

Use this "as is" or as a base for seasonings to make a sweet or savory dip. Soaked, drained almonds, allowed to sit in the refrigerator for a day or so, become soft enough to blend to a creamy consistency. If you can afford raw madacamia nuts, it will be more like dairy sour cream.

American		*Metric*
1 cup	Raw almonds, soaked overnight, drained and sprouted for 1–2 days in the refrigerator, or replace all or part of the almonds with rinsed macadamia nuts for a richer cream	140g
	Juice of 1 lemon	
	Water to blend	
	Unrefined salt to taste	
	For sweet dip: Add honey, stevia, and/or agave nectar to taste	
	For savory dip: Add shallots and chives	

Blend until smooth and creamy.

ALMOND CREAM CHEESE

Yes! You can eat this and not feel deprived.

1 recipe **Almond Sour Cream**

Place sour cream in a nut milk bag and hang over a bowl for 8–12 hours to catch the whey. Remove and refrigerate cheese. Use within a few days.

MOZZARELLA MACADAMIA

I first tasted this with summer fresh tomato slices as one course of a $100 a plate raw gourmet dinner. It was worth it to figure out how to make it for myself.

American		*Metric*
2 cups	Raw macadamia nuts	280g
	Water to blend	
	Juice of 1 lemon	
	1/2–1 teaspoon unrefined salt	
	Powdered thyme or Italian herbs	

Blend nuts and lemon juice with enough water to make a smooth, thick cream. Pour into a colander lined with several layers of cheesecloth or a nut milk bag over a bowl to catch the whey. Cover the colander or bowl with a cloth and let sit for 8–12 hours. Gently scrape cheese from cloth, form into a soft mass and refrigerate until needed. Sprinkle with powdered herbs and serve with **Give Us This Day Our Daily Bread Crackers** (see p. 86).

GOURMET RAW CANNELLONI

This indulgence can also be made with lower fat, and less expensive, soaked almonds or sunflower seeds substituting for the macadamia nuts.

2 medium zucchini (courgettes) or summer squash, sliced
very thin lengthwise with a mandoline

1 recipe **Morel Mushroom Brie** or
Macadamia Mozzarella (see above)

Place a small amount of brie filling at one end of a zucchini strip and roll up until it stays together. Trim end. Continue until filling is used. Place cannelloni on mesh sheets in a food dehydrator and dry for a few hours. Serve warm, plated with a puréed raw marinara sauce.

WALNUT PARM

Not quite the real thing but pretty darn close, considering the ingredients have nothing to do with cheese or the region of Parma, Italy. Use liberally on raw tomato dishes or as a salad sprinkle.

American		*Metric*
1 cup	Raw walnuts, soaked, rinsed and drained	140g
	3 tablespoons nutritional yeast	
	1 1/2 teaspoons unrefined salt	

Re-dry wet walnuts on mesh sheets of a dehydrator until thoroughly dry. Do not skip this step. Place dry nuts with yeast and salt in a food processor fitted with an "S" blade and pulse until it forms a grated cheese texture. Store in a capped container in refrigerator. It keeps a long time.

MOREL MUSHROOM BRIE

I created this just to see if it was possible to re-experience a fondly remembered cheese experience in a raw vegan incarnation. It was.

American		*Metric*
1 cup	Macadamia nuts, rinsed	140g
1/2 cup	Pine nuts, rinsed	70g
1 cup	Water or more as needed to blend	230ml
	Unrefined salt and pepper to taste	
1 cup	Dried morel mushrooms, crumbled	120g

Place nuts, salt, and pepper in blender with a portion of the water and blend, adding water in small amounts to keep the blender going until all is smooth. Adjust seasoning and finish by briefly blending in mushrooms, leaving small chunks. Pour into a nut milk bag or into a colander lined with several layers of cheesecloth and hang over a bowl for 8–12 hours. Scrape out cheese and shape into a soft brick. Slice or spread on crackers or use it to make cannelloni (see recipe below). Whey drippings can be added to soups or crackers if desired.

CHEESY SAUCE

Use this as a filling for **Cheese Dreams** (see p. 130) or over chopped vegetables.

American		Metric
	Juice of 1–2 lemons	
	1 tablespoon extra virgin olive oil	
	1 red bell pepper, chopped, with seeds	
	1 clove garlic	
	1 tablespoon Nama Shoyu or other unpasteurized soy sauce	
1 cup	Raw, hulled sunflower seeds, soaked several hours to overnight and drained	140g
1 cup	Raw almonds, soaked several hours to overnight, drained	140g
	Optional: Add 1 jalapeño to the mix for pepper cheese sauce	

Liquefy pepper and garlic in blender with lemon juice, olive oil, and soy sauce. Blend in seeds and almonds until smooth and creamy, adding water if necessary.

KEFIR LABNE

A vegan version of this creamy Middle Eastern staple.

American		Metric
1 quart	Almond milk kefir	1 litre
	1/2 teaspoon or more unrefined salt to taste	

Pour purchased or prepared kefir into a clean muslin or very fine meshed bag. Hang over a bowl to save the whey—a healthful drink all on its own. After 8–12 hours, scrape out the soft cheese, and then refrigerate or serve.

PESTO

This recipe provides more evidence that dairy cheese needn't be missed. Different varieties of basil will produce distinct, delicious variations. Use Genovese basil for a classic taste. Served over a plate of **Noodles al Dente** (see over), this makes a full meal or potluck dish.

American		*Metric*
	1 large bunch fresh basil, washed and chopped	
1/2 cup	Pine nuts, rinsed	70g
1/2 cup	Raw walnuts, soaked and re-dried, or unsoaked	70g
	2–3 cloves garlic	
1/2–1 cup	Extra virgin olive oil	115–230ml
	1/2–1 teaspoon unrefined salt or to taste	

Purée everything in a food processor fitted with an "S" blade or put through a Champion juicer with the blank plate.

THAI HAZELNUT PESTO

A refreshing alternative spread, less oily than the original version. Serve with crackers or **Noodles al Dente** (see over).

American		*Metric*
1 cup	Hazelnuts, soaked, drained and re-dried, or unsoaked	140g
	1 bunch mint, chopped	
	1 bunch cilantro (coriander leaf), chopped	
	1 bunch basil, chopped	
	3–4 cloves garlic	
	Juice of 3 lemons or limes	
1 cup	Extra virgin olive oil	230ml
	Unrefined salt and fresh ground black pepper to taste	

Purée everything in a food processor fitted with an "S" blade. This will keep in the refrigerator for a couple weeks.

RAW COPYCAT BURGER WITH FIXINGS

Great picnic fare and low carb, too! This recipe is an adaptation of the Boutenkos' raw gardenburger (www.rawfamily.com) and serves four to six as a main course.

To Make Burger

American		Metric
3 cups	Raw almonds, walnuts, or hazelnuts in any combination, soaked overnight and drained	420g
3 cups	Carrots, chopped	350g
	1 leek, chopped	
	Juice of 1 lemon	
1/4 cup	Extra virgin olive oil	60ml
	1–2 cloves garlic	
1/2 cup	Fresh mixed sage, oregano and thyme, chopped, or 3 tablespoons poultry seasoning	20g
	Unrefined salt to taste	
1/2 cup	Fresh ground flax seed meal	65g

Optional: Herbs such as rosemary and/or basil or jalapeño pepper

Place nuts in food processor fitted with an "S" blade and process to a coarse meal. Pour into large mixing bowl. Add carrots, leek, garlic, oil, herbs and salt to processor and process until well grated and mixed. Grind cup whole flax seeds in a spice grinder or dry blender. It will expand to cup. Process into carrot mix. Combine all of the above with nut meal and thoroughly mix with clean hands. Form patties and place on mesh dehydrator sheets to dry until crisp on the outside but still moist and chewy within. Small patties hold together better and dry faster.

To Assemble Fixings

3 vine ripe tomatoes, sliced

18–24 fairly large spinach leaves, de-stemmed

1 recipe **Almond Mayonnaise** (see p. 75)

Place 1 slice tomato on leaf, add patty and small amount of mayonnaise. Roll or fold over.

NOODLES AL DENTE

These are superior to their wheaten namesakes if turned out in a vegetable spiralizer or spirulli device. The spiralizer makes a fine angel hair or ribbon string noodle out of firm vegetables, while the spirulli spools out a continuous strand of thicker vermicelli in minutes. If you can't find one of these inexpensive hand-cranked gadgets in a specialty store or online, use the smallest julienne blade of a mandoline slicer, vegetable peeler, or your best knife technique.

1 or 2 medium zucchini (courgettes) or summer squash

As near as possible to serving, cut squash in half to fit a spiralizer or spirulli and process. Alternately, slice into thin ribbons with a vegetable peeler or knife.

RAW COPYCAT LASAGNA

It's one of my fussier recipes, but the result will please your friends, raw and non-raw alike. Plan ahead to soak nuts and make the ricotta cheese.

Raw Ricotta Layer

American		Metric
1 cup	Almonds, soaked a few hours to overnight and drained	140g
1 cup	Raw, hulled sunflower seeds, soaked a few hours to overnight and drained	140g
	Juice of 2 lemons	
	1 tablespoon extra virgin olive oil	
	Water to blend, if necessary	
	Unrefined salt and fresh ground black pepper to taste	

Blend everything together with as little water as possible. Pour into a colander lined with several layers of cheesecloth or a nut milk bag and hang over a bowl for a few hours to overnight. Gently squeeze out water.

Tomato Pesto Layer

American		Metric
1 cup	Dried tomatoes	140g
	Water to reconstitute	
	1 bunch basil	
1 cup	Pine nuts	140g
	2 cloves garlic	
1/4 cup	Extra virgin olive oil	60ml
	1/2 teaspoon unrefined salt	

Soften tomatoes in a small amount of water. Drain, reserving liquid, and place in a food processor fitted with an "S" blade. Pulse together with the rest of the ingredients until it is a thick paste. If need be, add enough of the tomato soak water to complete processing.

Mushroom Layer

American		Metric
	4 Portabello mushrooms	
1/4 cup	Nama Shoyu or other unpasteurized soy sauce	60ml

Rinse, dry, and stem caps. Slice thinly crosswise, place in bowl and stir in soy sauce to coat. Let sit hour to overnight in the refrigerator. Drain and press out excess liquid before using.

Vegetable Layers

1 bunch tender spinach, de-stemmed and chopped

3 medium zucchini (courgettes), sliced very thin lengthwise with a mandoline or vegetable peeler

2 vine ripe red tomatoes, sliced thin

Optional: 2 tablespoons **Walnut Parm** for garnish

To Assemble Lasagna

Lay strips of zucchini (courgette) lengthwise and then crosswise in a 9 x 12 inch glass casserole dish. Spoon some of the tomato pesto on top and spread evenly. Cover with a layer of spinach and then of the marinated mushroom slices. Spoon and spread some of the ricotta cheese on top. Repeat layers as before, ending with a final layer of zucchini (courgette) strips. Garnish with thin slices of fresh tomatoes and **Walnut Parm** (see p. 95). Warm in a food dehydrator for a few hours if it is large enough, or serve chilled.

RAW COPYCAT SPAGHETTI

Looks like spaghetti, smells like spaghetti, and tastes even better.

American		*Metric*
4 cups	Chopped vine, ripe tomatoes	520g
1/2 cup	Extra virgin olive oil	115ml
	2 chopped shallots	
	2 cloves garlic	
1/2–1 cup	Chopped fresh basil	50–100g
	1 tablespoon chopped fresh oregano	
	1 sprig fresh rosemary, stem removed	
	1/4–1/2 teaspoon cinnamon	
1 cup	Dried tomatoes	150g
	1 red bell pepper, chopped	
	Unrefined salt and fresh ground black pepper to taste	
	1 recipe **Noodles al Dente**, see above	
	1 recipe **Walnut Parm**	

Marinara Sauce: Place tomatoes, shallots, garlic, olive oil, bell pepper, herbs, and cinnamon in blender and blend until smooth. Add dried tomatoes and soften for an hour or so. Blend. Serve over **Noodles al Dente** with **Walnut Parm** (see p. 95).

TUNA PHISH ROLLS

Tuna salad was a staple of my childhood. This version brings back the memories.

American		Metric
4 cups	Raw walnuts, soaked several hours to overnight, drained and re-dried in refrigerator or dehydrator for a few hours	560g
1/2 cup	Apple cider vinegar	115ml
	Juice of 1 lemon	
1/2 cup	Extra virgin olive oil	115ml
	2 cups carrots, chopped	
	1 small onion, chopped	
	1 clove garlic	
1/2 cup	Parsley	20g
	Unrefined salt and fresh ground black pepper to taste	
2 cups	Celery, chopped	200g
	1 package raw (untoasted) nori sheets	

Place walnuts in dry food processor fitted with an "S" blade and pulse to small chunks. Pour into a large mixing bowl. Purée carrots, onion, and garlic with liquids. Pulse in celery, parsley, and seasonings. Thoroughly mix in bowl with the nuts. On a dry surface with dry hands, spread out a sheet of nori. Place a thick line of filling mix across the width of the nori and roll up snugly. Seal by dipping a finger in water, running it along the edge and then pressing together. Cut into rolls with a sharp knife and place on a nice plate. Refrigerate until served. Note: nori wrappers will quickly soften, so don't make these too far ahead unless you want to eat them with a fork instead of as a finger food.

CHAPTER 8

FEAST FOOD

A delightful entrée for many of us into the raw food world was being invited to a meal or party featuring raw gourmet dishes. On such occasions the community-building blessing of eating together is doubled by the quality and value of the food. It's fun, too. I love being introduced to a new dish and then going home to try it out myself.

Becoming a fine raw chef is not that difficult, and just mastering a few favorite preparations is even easier. Remember **Jim's Signature Salad** (see p. 68) that he takes everywhere and eats at home as well. If you've read this far, you already have a good sense of the basic techniques. This chapter offers menus based around some of my favorite entrées and suggestions for raw buffet spreads.

RAW MEX MENU

Here are some empowered versions of Mexican favorites to serve together or alone.

Guacamole

4 ripe avocados, chopped

2 cloves garlic

2–3 green onions, chopped

Juice of 2 lemons or limes

1–2 jalapenos, with seeds, chopped

Optional: 1 bunch cilantro (coriander leaf)

Unrefined salt or Nama Shoyu soy sauce, to taste

Pulse everything together in a food processor fitted with an "S" blade to your preferred consistency.

Fresh Salsa

American		Metric
	4–6 vine ripe tomatoes, chopped	
	1 red bell pepper, chopped	
	1 onion	
	3 cloves garlic	
	1 bunch cilantro (coriander leaf)	
1/4 cup	Raw apple cider vinegar	60ml
	1–2 jalapenos with seeds, chopped	
1/2 cup	Dried tomatoes	60g
	Unrefined salt to taste	

Blend everything but dried tomatoes together in a blender or food processor. Stir in dried tomatoes and allow to soften for about an hour. Finish blending.

Corn Crackers

American		Metric
1 cup	Golden flax seed	140g
1 cup	Water	230ml
	2 fresh ears of corn	
	1 tablespoon extra virgin olive oil	
	1–2 teaspoons unrefined salt, or to taste	
	Optional: add 1 jalapeño with seeds	

Rinse flax seed in a strainer. Cut corn off the cobs. Place corn and flax in blender with water, salt, and olive oil. Blend until seeds are broken up. Wait a few minutes to thicken and then spread onto mesh sheets of dehydrator to dry until crisp.

Chili Raw

American		Metric
	2 ripe tomatoes, chopped	
	2 cloves garlic	
1/4 cup	Raisins	35g
	2 tablespoons extra virgin olive oil	
	1 tablespoon chili powder	
1 cup	Dried tomatoes	120g
	Unrefined salt to taste	
2 cups	Raw walnuts, soaked and drained	280g
1 cup	Raw, hulled sunflower seeds, soaked a few hours to overnight, rinsed and drained	140g
	2 fresh ears of corn, cut off the cob	
	1 red bell pepper, chopped	

Purèe tomatoes in blender or food processor with garlic, raisins, olive oil, and chili powder. Stir in dried tomatoes and allow to soften. Blend. Add salt and more chili powder to taste. Place walnuts, bell pepper, and sunflower seeds in a food processor fitted with an "S" blade and pulse until roughly chopped. Stir in tomato mixture and corn.

Burrito Wraps

1 recipe **Fresh Salsa**

1 recipe **Chili Raw**

1 recipe **Guacamole**

Spinach, collard, chard or kale leaves, trimmed to use as wraps

Place a small amount of chili filling on each wrap and roll into a burrito. Serve with **Fresh Salsa** (see p. 106), **Guacamole** (see p. 105) and **Almond Sour Cream** (see p. 93), if desired.

SWEDISH NEATBALL DINNER

Cooked folks are surprised to see these, and even more surprised at how good they taste. Use them as a finger food for a potluck or buffet or to make a meal accompanied by a green salad and fresh sauerkraut. You can use the **Copycat Burger** recipe (see p. 98) to make the neatballs or this variation with sunflower seeds.

American		*Metric*
	Neatballs	
2 cups	Raw walnuts, almonds, or hazelnuts, soaked a few hours to overnight and drained	280g
1 cup	Raw, hulled sunflower seeds, soaked a few hours to overnight and drained	140g
2 cups	Carrots, chopped	220g
	1 leek or onion	
	2 tablespoons raw apple cider vinegar	
	2 tablespoons extra virgin olive oil	
1/2 cup	Fresh ground flax seed meal	70g
	Poultry seasoning or fresh herbs such as sage, rosemary, thyme, parsley, oregano, or marjoram to taste	
	Unrefined salt and fresh ground black pepper to taste	
	Sweet and Sour Sauce	
1/2 cup	Raw apple cider vinegar	115ml
1/2 cup	Nama Shoyu or other unpasteurized soy sauce	115ml
	1 tablespoon extra virgin olive oil	
	1 tablespoon raw honey or agave nectar or to taste	
	2 cloves garlic	
2 cups	Dried tomatoes	200g
	1 apple or pear, chopped	

Place nuts and sunflower seeds in food processor fitted with an "S" blade and process to a coarse meal. Pour into large mixing bowl. Add carrots, onion, garlic, oil, herbs, and salt and process until well grated and mixed. Grind 1/2 cup (70g) whole flax seeds in a spice grinder or dry blender. It will expand to cup. Process into carrot mix. Combine everything with nut meal and thoroughly mix with clean hands.

Roll mix into small balls and place on mesh dehydrator sheets for several hours. Dry until firm on the outside.

For the sauce, place liquids in a blender with the apple and garlic and purée. Add tomatoes and immerse in liquid. Let sit at least an hour to soften. Purée when soft. Dip warm neatballs in sauce and return to dehydrator for an hour to firm up coating if using as a finger food. Serve with remaining sauce.

SHEPHERD'S PIE

This is another recipe courtesy of Rosi Goldsmith. She created this one-dish meal as an offering for a new mother and found lots of other takers.

Crust

American		Metric
1 cup	Sprouted buckwheat	120g
2 cups	Sprouted, soaked sunflower seeds	240g
2 cups	Golden flax seed, soaked	280g
	1 tablespoon dried dill or 3 tablespoons fresh	
	Unrefined salt to taste	

Process all ingredients in a food processor fitted with the "S" blade until smooth. Spread very thinly, about 3/16 inch, and dehydrate until dry and still pliable but not crisp.

Filling

American		Metric
	2 large celery stalks	
	2 carrots, grated	
	2 beets, grated	
2 cups	Cauliflower, grated	240g
	1/3 to 1/2 head broccoli	
	1/2 bunch fresh kale	
	1 small leek	
	1/2 zucchini (courgette)	

Slice vegetables thinly and marinate in **Cream Sauce**, below. To assemble, layer crust pieces to cover a pie plate. Alternate green layers, grated beets, grated cauliflower and grated carrots. Add filling layers with beets and carrots on top and pour the rest of the sauce over.

Cream Sauce

American		Metric
2 cups	Combined, soaked, and sprouted sunflower and hazelnuts	280g
2 cups	Sprouted mung beans, or lentils sprouted for 3 days	260g
	3 tablespoons fresh thyme	
	1 1/2 tablespoons fresh sage	
	1 1/2 tablespoons dried Italian herbs	
	Juice of one large or 2 medium lemons	
1/4 cup	Olive oil	60ml
	Unrefined salt to taste	
1/2–1 cup	Water to desired thickness	115–230ml

Mix in the blender.

MEZZA PLATE

One of the first things I tried to make in a raw version was the hummus of fond memory. It became a staple my first raw year because it was so filling and lasted well in the refrigerator. Hummus becomes falafel with a few extra touches and some time in the dehydrator. I also tried several raw tabouli salads made with different sprouted grains and decided they tasted better without the grains. To round out your mezza plate, serve with **Zaatar Crisps** (see p. 86) and black olives.

Hummus

American		*Metric*
2 cups	Dried garbanzo beans (chick peas), soaked overnight and sprouted for 2–3 days	280g
1 cup	Brown, unhulled, raw sesame seeds, soaked for several hours to overnight, rinsed and drained	140g
	1 bunch parsley, chopped	
	2–3 stalks celery, chopped	
	Juice of 3–4 lemons	
1/2–1 cup	Extra virgin olive oil	115–230ml
	1–2 teaspoons unrefined salt or to taste	

This can be made in a Champion juicer with the blank plate or in a blender. Using a blender requires a larger amount of olive oil or additional water to blend smoothly. To make in a Champion, alternate ingredients and push through the funnel. Put the hummus through a second time to make it smoother. To use a blender, place liquid ingredients, salt, celery, and parsley together and liquefy. Add sesame seeds and blend. Add garbanzos (chick peas) in small amounts through the open top with blender running and carefully push down with a rubber spatula. If your blender is small, halve recipe or make in two batches.

Tabouli Salad

American		Metric
	3 vine ripe tomatoes, diced	
	2 cucumbers, diced	
	1 bunch parsley	
	1 bunch mint	
	1–2 tablespoons fresh oregano or 1 tablespoon dried	
	Juice of 1–2 lemons	
1/4 cup	Extra virgin olive oil	60ml
	Unrefined salt to taste	
	Optional:	
1/2 cup	Pitted olives, chopped	60g

Pulse parsley, mint, oregano, lemon juice, olive oil, and salt in a food processor fitted with an "S" blade. Stir into diced tomatoes and cucumbers.

Falafel

American		Metric
	1 recipe **Hummus** (see next page)	
1/2 cup	Fresh ground flax seed meal	70g
	1 teaspoon ground cumin	
	2 teaspoons ground coriander	
	1–2 tablespoons extra virgin olive oil	

Mix everything together thoroughly in a large bowl. Form into small balls and place on mesh dehydrator sheets to dry several hours to overnight until firm.

Raw-Ba-Ghanoush

John Larsen, raw chef extraordinaire (orderrawfood@vegemail.com) has brilliantly solved the problem of how to use raw eggplant (aubergine) in this tasty dish!

American		Metric
4 cups	Eggplant (aubergine), chopped	600g
	4 cloves garlic	
1 cup	Raw sesame tahini	150g
1/3 cup	Olive oil	90ml
	1 lemon, juiced	
1/2 cup	Parsley, chopped	20g
	salt to taste	
	1/2 teaspoon pepper	

Freeze the chopped eggplant (aubergine) for 24 hours to soften. Defrost for 2 hours. Place the eggplant (aubergines) in the food processor and pulse for 30 seconds. Add the remainder of the ingredients and process until creamy. Use as a dip or spread.

Kabees El Lift

American		Metric
	1 turnip	
	1 beet	
	2 cloves garlic, crushed	
1/2 cup	Apple cider vinegar	115ml
	1/2–1 teaspoon unrefined salt, or to taste	

Peel beet and turnip and slice into small pieces. Place in a jar with garlic, vinegar and salt. Cover, shake, and store in refrigerator. It will keep several weeks.

Dolmades

American		Metric
1 cup	Pine nuts, rinsed	140g
1 cup	Raw, hulled sunflower seeds, soaked a few hours to overnight, rinsed and drained	140g
1 cup	Whole barley, soaked overnight, drained and sprouted for 2 days	140g
	Juice of 2 lemons	
	1 clove garlic	
1 cup	Fresh mint leaves	80g
1/2 cup	Parsley, chopped	40g
	1 tablespoon extra virgin olive oil	
	Unrefined salt and fresh ground black pepper to taste	
	Spinach leaves or tender young grape leaves, de-stemmed	

Pulse all ingredients in a food processor fitted with an "S" blade until they stick together but still have some individuality. Pick grape leaves when young or from the end of the vines. Alternatively, harvest when tender and store in freezer in ziplock bags until needed. You can also try marinating more mature ones in lemon juice and salt for a day or so in the refrigerator. Spinach leaves also work great. Put a small amount of filling on each leaf. Roll, tuck in ends and serve, or warm in dehydrator before serving if desired.

GINGER BEET PICKLES

American		Metric
	2–3 pieces fresh ginger, peeled and sliced thin	
	1 small beet, peeled and sliced	
1/2 cup	Apple cider vinegar	115ml
	teaspoon unrefined salt	

Pack a small jar with ginger and beet slices. Add vinegar and salt, cap tightly and shake. Keeps in refrigerator for weeks.

CURRIED LENTIL CROQUETTES WITH RAISIN CHUTNEY

Serve this with **Coriander Raita** (see p. 66) and **Fruit Chat Masala** (see p. 74) for an Indian-inspired dinner.

Lentil Croquettes

American		Metric
2 cups	Sprouted lentils	200g
1 cup	Raw, hulled sunflower seeds, soaked several hours to overnight, drained and rinsed	140g
1/2 cup	Extra virgin olive oil	115ml
	3 cloves garlic	
	1–2 tablespoons cumin powder	
	Unrefined salt or Nama Shoyu to taste	
1/2 cup	Fresh ground flax seed meal	65g

Mix lentils, sunflower seeds, olive oil, garlic, cumin, and salt together in a food processor with an "S" blade until blended. Pulse in flax seed meal. Let sit briefly until it becomes thick enough to form patties. Dry patties on the mesh sheet of a food dehydrator for several hours until outside is crisp. Serve with **Raisin Chutney** and **Curry Sauce** (see below).

Raisin Chutney

American		Metric
1 cup	Raisins, soaked	140g
	1 apple or pear, chopped	
	1 jalapeño , chopped, with seeds	
	1 tablespoon fresh ginger, chopped	
	1 tablespoon fresh orange peel, chopped	
	2 teaspoons garam masala spice	
	Unrefined salt to taste	

Pulse everything together in a food processor fitted with the "S" blade.

Curry Sauce

American		Metric
2 cups	Winter squash, peeled and chopped	240g
	2 red bell peppers, chopped	
	Juice of 1 orange	
	2 tablespoons fresh ginger, chopped	
	2 tablespoons unrefined coconut oil	
	1–2 tablespoons curry powder	
	Unrefined salt to taste	

Liquefy bell peppers with orange juice, ginger, curry powder, salt, and oil in a blender. Blend in winter squash until smooth.

SUSHI FUSION

Sushi didn't appeal to me before I went raw except for the pickled ginger and wasabi sauce on the side. But nori can be wrapped around any salad, paté, or combination of shredded vegetables for a raw finger food.

5 sheets untoasted, dried nori

2 avocados, sliced

1 apple, sliced thin

2 carrots, sliced lengthwise into long matchsticks

1 recipe **Chili Raw** (see p. 107)

Lay nori out one sheet at a time on a dry surface. Spread a thick line of chili paste from end to end across the width nearest you. Cover with apple slices, carrot matchsticks, and avocado slices. Roll snugly and seal by dipping a finger in water, running it along the edge and then pressing together. Hold roll at one end and slice into rounds with a sharp knife. Serve with **Wasabi Sauce** (see p. 64) and **Ginger Beet Pickles** (p. 114) or **Fresh Salsa** (see p. 106).

TASTE OF CHINA

Have some more fun with your noodle-making gadgets to create this improvement over ramen.

American		*Metric*
1/4 cup	Nama Shoyu or other unpasteurized soy sauce	60ml
1/4 cup	Unrefined cold pressed sesame oil	60ml
1/4 cup	Raw apple cider vinegar	60ml
	1–2 teaspoons raw honey or agave nectar to taste	
	1 tablespoon fresh ginger, minced	
	2 cloves garlic, minced	
	2 firm zucchini (courgettes) or summer squash	
	1 small lotus root	
	12 fresh water chestnuts	
	1 tablespoon brown or black sesame seeds, soaked a few hours to overnight, rinsed and drained	

Optional: cup dried sea vegetable pieces, your choice, reconstituted in water and drained

Variation: Use sweet potato, kohlrabi or rutabaga (swede) for some or all of the noodles

Make sauce first by combining soy sauce, oil, vinegar, sweetener, garlic, and ginger in a bowl. Make noodles with the zucchini (courgettes) or summer squash, and stir into sauce. Peel lotus root and slice thinly across its width with a mandoline or sharp knife. Stir into sauce. Peel water chestnuts, chop if desired and add to sauce. Stir in optional sea vegetables and sprinkle with sesame seeds.

COMFORT AND JOY

After traveling for a month and subsisting on very plain raw food, this was the first thing I wanted upon my return.

American		Metric
1 cup	Brazil nuts, rinsed	140g
1 cup	Pine nuts, rinsed	140g
	Juice of 2 lemons	
1/4 cup	Extra virgin olive oil	60ml

1 tablespoon Chinese 5-spice blend or
make your own with 1 teaspoon cloves, 1 teaspoon cinnamon
and 1 teaspoon ground fennel seeds

Water as needed to blend

Unrefined salt to taste

2 heads cauliflower or broccoli, chopped into bite
size chunks, tough stems peeled first.

Place everything except chopped vegetables in blender and blend until creamy. Mix in a large bowl with vegetables to coat. Dry on mesh sheets for several hours and serve warm with **Half Naked Tomatoes**, below.

HALF NAKED TOMATOES

4–6 vine ripe tomatoes, sliced
Unrefined salt and fresh ground black pepper
1 tablespoon balsamic vinegar

Sprinkle tomatoes with salt, pepper, and vinegar. Say thanks.

SPROUT PIE
WITH STUFFED MUSHROOMS

American		*Metric*
2 cups	Small sprouts such as alfalfa or clover	200g
	2 vine ripe tomatoes, diced	
	1 recipe **Pesto** or **Thai Hazelnut Pesto** (see p. 97)	

Cover the bottom of a glass pie plate with half of the sprouts. Cover that with half of the pesto. Spread diced tomatoes on top and cover with remaining pesto. Press remaining sprouts on top and invert pie plate over a serving plate. Serve with **Stuffed Mushrooms**, below.

STUFFED MUSHROOMS

American		*Metric*
	20–24 small to medium crimini mushrooms	
2 cups	Raw walnuts, soaked a few hours to overnight, rinsed and drained	280g
1/2 cup	Pine nuts, rinsed	70g
	1 tablespoon extra virgin olive oil	
	1 tablespoon Nama Shoyu or other unpasteurized soy sauce	
	2 cloves garlic	
	2 tablespoons fresh sage, chopped, or 2 teaspoons poultry seasoning	
	1 tablespoon nutritional yeast	
	Unrefined salt and fresh ground black pepper to taste	

Quickly rinse mushrooms, drain, and set aside. Remove stems. Place stems, along with the other ingredients, in a food processor fitted with an "S" blade and process to a paste. Fill mushroom caps and place stuffing side up on mesh trays in a food dehydrator to warm and dry for several hours before serving.

WILD MUSHROOM TART

Chanterelles are hidden treasures in the summer woods. Morels greet lucky seekers in the spring. Whenever you find some in the woods or market, dry them for this special treat. The rich filling uses only a minimum of seasonings to allow the delicate mushroom flavor to shine. Serve with mâche or other mild greens and **Raspberry Vinaigrette** (see p. 63).

Crust

American		*Metric*
2 cups	Walnuts, soaked a few hours to overnight, rinsed and drained	280g
	1/2 teaspoon unrefined salt	

Process to a crumbly paste in a food processor fitted with an "S" blade. Press into a glass pie plate. Place in food dehydrator for 4–8 hours to dry.

Filling

American		*Metric*
	1 tablespoon agar-agar or kosher gelatin flakes	
1/2 cup	Water	115ml
2 cups	Shelled, raw macadamia nuts, rinsed	280g
	1 small shallot	
1 cup	Dried chanterelles, morels, or porcini in small pieces	90g
	Unrefined salt and fresh ground black pepper to taste	

Dissolve agar-agar in hot water and put in blender. Add macadamia nuts and shallot. Blend to a thick cream, using the least possible amount of added water. Blend in mushroom pieces and seasonings and pour into prepared crust. Warm in a dehydrator for several hours before serving.

VEGETABLES EXCALIBUR

A simple presentation of warm marinated vegetables dressed up with tasty **Cheese Dreams** (see p. 129). A good combo to make when red bell peppers are in season.

American		Metric
	2–4 red bell peppers	
	1–2 zucchini(courgette) or other soft squash	
	1 sweet onion	
2 cups	Mushrooms	150g
	1 head broccoli	
	2 carrots	
	Optional: 2 apples for a surprising sweet bite	
1/4 cup	Extra virgin olive oil	60ml
1/2 cup	Raw apple cider vinegar	115ml
1/2 cup	Nama Shoyu or other unpasteurized soy sauce	115ml
	4 cloves garlic, minced	

Chop vegetables, with optional apple, into bite-size pieces and place in a large bowl. Mix oil, vinegar, and soy sauce with garlic and mix in with vegetables, stirring to coat. Cover and marinate for several hours to overnight, stirring occasionally. Place marinated vegetables on dehydrator trays and dry for several hours or longer. Serve warm accompanied with **Cheese Dreams** (see p. 129) for a satisfying dinner.

HURRAW FOR THE PUMPKIN PIE
THANKSGIVING DINNER

Raw vegans needn't fear or avoid this traditional meal laden with so many family associations. Carry some of these dishes with you over the river and through the woods to grandmother's house. You could just eat the pumpkin pie and have a great nourishing meal. Next year, invite everybody to your place, bringing their own turkey if they feel the need.

Stuffed Portabellos with Mushroom Gravy

American		Metric
	6 matching Portabello mushrooms	
1/2 cup	Nama Shoyu or other unpasteurized soy sauce	115ml
1/2 cup	Extra virgin olive oil	115ml
	2 cloves garlic, minced	
2 cups	Raw walnuts, soaked a few hours to overnight, rinsed and drained	280g
	1 onion, diced	
	6 stalks celery, chopped	
	3 carrots, chopped	
1 cup	Pine nuts, rinsed	140g
	1 apple, chopped	
	1 tablespoon poultry seasoning plus fresh sage, thyme, parsley, and rosemary or use more poultry seasoning	
	1/2–1 teaspoon unrefined salt and fresh ground black pepper, to taste	

Quickly rinse and pat dry mushrooms. Remove stems and marinate in olive oil and soy sauce while assembling the filling. Pulse walnuts until chopped in a food processor fitted with an "S" blade. Pour into a large mixing bowl. Combine mushroom stems, pine nuts, apple, onion, carrots, celery, garlic, and seasonings in food processor and blend thoroughly. Mix in with walnuts. Drain mushroom caps, fill with stuffing, and place on mesh dehydrator trays for 4–8 hours. To serve, press two mushroom halves together and set on a platter ringed with **Fresh Cranberry Sauce** and topped with **Mushroom Gravy** (see below).

Mushroom Gravy

American		Metric
	Any remaining marinade from above recipe	
1/2 cup	Nama Shoyu or other unpasteurized soy sauce	115ml
1/2 cup	Extra virgin olive oil	115ml
1/4 cup	Water	60ml
	1 shallot	
	1 clove garlic	
	2 tablespoons powdered dried shiitake, porcini or wild mushrooms	
1/4 cup	Pine nuts, rinsed	35g

Blend everything together in a blender until smooth.

Fresh Cranberry Sauce

American		Metric
2 cups	Fresh cranberries, rinsed	260g
	2 soft ripe pears, seeded and chopped	
1/4–1/2 cup	Raw honey or agave nectar with stevia extract powder, to taste	60–120g
	1/2 teaspoon nutmeg	
	1/2 teaspoon cinnamon	
	Unrefined salt to taste	

Optional: Replace spices with 1 teaspoon fresh minced thyme

Combine all in a food processor fitted with an "S" blade and process until completely blended.

Hurraw For the Pumpkin Pie

See p. 131.

A RAW BUFFET

Raw gourmet is really party food to be shared. **Swedish Neatballs** (see p. 108), **Stuffed Mushrooms** (see p. 119), and **Cheese Dreams** (see p. 129) are all ready to go. Here are some more ideas for what to offer as appetizers and finger foods.

Taste of Olive Tapenade

American		Metric
	2 large, red bell peppers, seeded, chopped, and dried until pliable	
1/2 cup	Pitted, Kalamata olives	65g
	1 teaspoon extra virgin olive oil	
	Optional but heavenly: Use truffle-infused olive oil	

Chop everything together in a food processor fitted with an "S" blade or by hand. Spread on crackers or use as a dip.

RV Rumakis

RV stands for raw vegan. In their original incarnation, Rumakis were made with chicken livers. This unusual version of a Tiki bar favorite is guaranteed to help start conversations around your party buffet.

American		Metric
	24 prunes	
1/2 cup	Nama Shoyu or other unpasteurized soy sauce	115ml
1/2 cup	Raw apple cider vinegar	115ml
	2 tablespoons fresh ginger, chopped	
	24 fresh water chestnuts	

Cover prunes with soy sauce, ginger, and vinegar and soak overnight. Remove pits. Peel water chestnuts and stuff inside prunes.

Pesto Dabs

1 recipe **Pesto**, any type (see p. 87)

Cherry tomatoes

Cut cherry tomatoes in half, dab with pesto, and arrange on a platter. These go fast at a party.

Pizza Rolls

From raw chef John Larsen (orderrawfood@vegemail.com).

American		Metric
2 cups	Sun dried tomatoes, soaked 1 hour	300g
2 cups	Packed fresh basil	120g
3 cups	Walnuts, soaked 6 hours	420g
	6 cloves garlic, crushed	
	1 tablespoon olive oil	
	2 tablespoons water from soaking the tomatoes	
	1 tablespoon freshly ground black pepper	
	1/2 lemon, juiced	
	1 teaspoon unprocessed salt or to taste	
	5 zucchini squash	

Mix all ingredients, except the zucchini, in a food processor. Process into a smooth paste. Using a vegetable peeler slice zucchini lengthwise. Cut these strips in half crosswise to create 4" strips. Place a small amount of paste onto a strip of zucchini and roll up. Place these bite-sized rolls onto a dehydrator tray and dehydrate until firm. Enjoy!

Antipasto Vegetables and Dip

Selection of attractively cut raw vegetables: Along with the usual carrots, celery, radish, and cucumbers, consider asparagus, jicama, corn on the cob broken into thin wheels with a cleaver, snow peas, string beans, winter squash, sweet potatoes, kohlrabi, rutabaga (swede), yacon, and the like. Arrange sumptuously on a platter with bowls of dip nearby. Use any sauce, dressing, or dip recipes that appeal, or create your own using soaked nuts or seeds in any combination with oil, lemon juice, or apple cider vinegar and your favorite herbs.

Buffet Fruit Platter

Selection of seasonal and exotic fruits: Consider grapes, strawberries, cherries, pineapple, melons, Asian pears, pomegranate, kiwi, apples, yacon, and oranges. Prepare some for dipping and leave others, such as tangerines, rambutans, lychees, and finger bananas, for guests to peel. Serve with **Amazing Avocado Icing and Fruit Fondue** (see p. 51), **Sweet Fennel Seed Dressing** (see p. 64) or your own creations.

RAW PARTY DRINKS

The main issue here is raw drinks are so nourishing that you don't need to eat much, if anything, for at least a few hours. I always offer filtered water to guests before meals. After eating, I offer iced or hot herbal teas. Yes, I know that's not raw. You can make a raw sun tea with some herbs if you have time. For me, the benefits of the herbs and the increased possibility of social sharing that comes with at least being an herbal tea drinker outweigh any other costs in my mind. You decide. Meanwhile, here are some other great drinks to try.

Fruit Nog

American		Metric
2 cups	**Raw Almond Milk** (see p. 52)	460ml
	1–2 soft ripe pears	
	1 ripe banana	
	1 teaspoon vanilla or vanilla bean	
	1/2 teaspoon nutmeg	
	Sprinkle of unrefined salt	
	Stevia, raw honey or agave nectar, to taste	
Blend and serve.		

Beetgrass Juice

1–2 beets, chopped

2–3 carrots, chopped

1 apple, chopped

1 tablespoon fresh ginger, chopped

Handful of wheatgrass

Handful of fresh mint

Put everything through the funnel of a Samson juicer, or juice everything else in most other juicers and leave out the wheatgrass.

Chai

American		Metric
	6 cardamom pods or 1 teaspoon hulled seeds	
	1 tablespoon coriander seeds, crushed	
	1–3 teaspoons dried licorice root, cut or chopped	
3 cups	Water	690ml
3 cups	Raw almonds, soaked a few hours to overnight, rinsed and drained	420g
	2 teaspoons powdered cinnamon	
	Optional: 1/2 teaspoon vanilla	

Brew cardamom, coriander, and licorice root with boiled water in a non-metal pot. Let stand until cool. Strain out herbs and use liquid to make almond milk by blending with soaked nuts. Strain out pulp or leave in as desired. Add more water for a thinner chai. Warm gently and serve in warmed mugs with cinnamon sprinkled on top.

Avo Shake

Water and meat of 1 green coconut

2 ripe avocados, peeled and seeded

Juice of 1–2 limes

Stevia extract powder, raw honey or agave nectar, to taste

Blend and serve chilled.

Water in the Shell

1 green coconut per guest

1 straw per coconut

Remove husk from the pointed end by scoring a circle with a sharp knife and prying off, exposing the thin flesh. Poke a straw through this and serve. For dessert, have a cleaver handy to split nuts in half when guests have drunk all the water, and then provide spoons to scoop out the meat.

VISHNU'S PATE

This recipe courtesy of John Larsen (orderrawfood@vegemail.com). Delicious with **Chappati Bread** (see p. 88).

American		*Metric*
2 cups	Walnuts	280g
	1 medium sweet onion, chopped	
	4 stalks celery, chopped	
	2–3 carrots	
	1 tablespoon raw honey	
1/2 cup	Extra-virgin olive oil	115ml
	1/4 teaspoon poultry seasoning	
	1/2 teaspoon curry powder	
	1 1/2 teaspoon turmeric	

Place walnuts in processor and pulse into a granular consistency, set aside. Place onion, celery and carrots in processor and process until granular. Add the walnuts back into the processor along with the oil, honey and spices and process until creamy.

LIVING FUDGE

This only takes a few minutes to make and the surprise ingredient will not be guessed.

American		Metric
3 cups	Shredded dried coconut	
1/2 cup	Raw carob powder	70g
1 cup	Alfalfa sprouts	100g
1/3 cup	Raw honey or agave nectar	90g
	1 teaspoon vanilla	

Process coconut with carob, honey and vanilla until mixed. Add sprouts and process until it forms a clump. Press into a pan at desired thickness and chill before cutting into squares.

CHEESE MELT

Here's another cheesy sauce with some different ingredients to try. This one is nice with tomatoes and avocados.

American		Metric
1/2 cup	Pine nuts, rinsed	70g
1/2–1 cup	Raw almonds or raw, unhulled sunflower seeds, soaked, rinsed and drained	70–140g
1/4 cup	Extra virgin olive oil	60ml
	Juice of 1 lemon	
	2 tablespoons white or mellow miso, unpasteurized	
	1 tablespoon turmeric powder	
	1 teaspoon onion powder	
	1/2 teaspoon freshly ground black pepper	
	Optional for nacho cheese: 1/2–1 whole jalapeño pepper	

Place all ingredients except nuts and seeds in a blender and liquefy. Blend in pine nuts, then almonds or sunflower seeds until smooth, adding a small amount of water to blender if necessary.

CHEESE DREAMS

American		Metric
	Juice of 1–2 lemons	
1/4 cup	Nama Shoyu or other unpasteurized soy sauce	60ml
	1 red bell pepper, chopped	
	3 cloves garlic	
1/2 cup	Raw almonds, soaked a few hours to overnight, rinsed and drained	70g
1/2 cup	Raw, hulled sunflower seeds, soaked a few hours to overnight, rinsed and drained	70g
1 cup	Pine nuts, rinsed	140g
	1 jicama, peeled	
	Optional for Pepper Cheese Dreams: 1 jalapeño	

Liquefy bell pepper and garlic with lemon juice and Nama Shoyu in a blender. Blend in almonds, sunflower seeds, and pine nuts to a thick paste. Use a mandoline to create very thin slices from the jicama, the consistency of wonton wrappers. Place a teaspoon of the paste on one side of each slice and fold over to make a wrap. These may be served "as is" or warmed in a dehydrator for an hour or so.

CHAPTER 9

SWEET FOOD

RAW PIES

One of the secrets of raw pies is the crust, of course, and raw pie crusts, especially the dessert ones, can be so simple. In most cases use soaked and re-dried nuts or unsoaked if you didn't plan ahead. Wet nuts work when drying the crust separately from the filling. The other main ingredient is some kind of dried fruit for sweetness and stickiness. Dates and raisins are the most common choices, but try figs, apricots, or prunes for a different treatment. Raw honey or agave nectar may replace all or some of the fruit for a very sweet crust.

HURRAW FOR THE PUMPKIN PIE

Crust

American		*Metric*
3 cups	Raw walnuts, hazelnuts, or almonds in any combination, soaked, rinsed and re-dried, or unsoaked	420g
1 1/2 cups	Raisins or pitted dates, rinsed	210g
	Sprinkle of unprocessed salt	

Chop nuts in a food processor fitted with an "S" blade. Add fruit and salt, and then blend to a sticky dough. Press into a 9–10 inch non-metal pie plate.

Filling

American		Metric
	2 tablespoons agar-agar or kosher gelatin flakes	
1/2 cup	Water	115ml
3–4 cups	Raw pumpkin or winter squash, peeled, seeded, and chopped	300–400g
1/4–1/2 cup	Raw honey or agave nectar	60–120g
	1 tablespoon fresh ginger, minced	
	1 teaspoon vanilla	
	1 tablespoon pumpkin pie spice	
1 cup	Fresh macadamia nuts, rinsed	140g
	Sprinkle of unprocessed salt	

Optional: Substitute 1 tablespoon psyllium seed husk powder for the agar and omit water. Pie will have a less custardy texture but still taste the same.

Dissolve agar-agar in hot water, and then process with the pumpkin, vanilla, ginger, and honey in a food processor fitted with an "S" blade until blended. Transfer to a blender and liquefy further. Add spice, salt, nuts, and, if using, psyllium. Blend to a thick custard and pour into prepared crust. Chill, partially freeze, or warm in a dehydrator before serving. Serve with **Cream Whip** (see below) for added glory.

Cream Whip

American		Metric
1 1/2 cups	Raw macadamia nuts, rinsed	210g
1/2 cup	Pine nuts, rinsed	70g
	Juice of 1 orange	
	Juice of 1 lemon	
	1 teaspoon vanilla or 1 inch vanilla bean	
1/4 cup	Raw honey or agave nectar, with stevia extract powder, to taste	60g
	Sprinkle unrefined salt	

Blend in a blender until creamy.

MOM'S APPLE PIE

Crust

American		Metric
3 cups	Raw walnuts, hazelnuts, or almonds in any combination, soaked and rinsed	420g
1 1/2 cup	Raisins or pitted dates, rinsed	210g
	Sprinkle of unrefined salt	

Chop nuts in a food processor fitted with an "S" blade. Add fruit and salt and blend to a sticky dough. Press into a 9–10 inch non-metal pie plate.

Filling

American		Metric
	6 large, good-tasting apples	
1/2 cup	Dried figs, chopped	70g
	Juice of 1 lemon	
1/4 cup	Raw honey or agave nectar, or to taste	60g
	1 tablespoon pumpkin pie spice	
	Sprinkle unrefined salt	

Core and cut four of the apples into small, thin slices. A food processor slicing blade does this in moments. Place in prepared crust. Core and chop remaining two apples and put in a food processor fitted with an "S" blade along with the rest of the ingredients. Blend to a thick slurry. Pour over apples in crust and stir in gently. Place pie in a food dehydrator for 4–8 hours to warm and soften apples. Serve warm with **Macadamia Nut Ice Cream** (see p. 153) or **Frozen Banana Soft Serve** (see p. 154) if desired.

APPLE CRISP

American		Metric
	6–8 apples	
	Juice of 2 lemons	
1/2 cup	Raw honey or agave nectar	100g
	Sprinkle of unrefined salt	
3 cups	Raw walnuts	420g
	1 tablespoon pumpkin pie spice	
	1 teaspoon cinnamon	
	1 teaspoon vanilla	

Core and cut apples into small, thin slices with a food processor slicing blade or a knife. Place in a glass or ceramic dish that fits in your dehydrator. Mix lemon juice, half the honey, and salt, and then stir into apple slices. Combine nuts, remaining honey, vanilla, and spices in a food processor fitted with an "S" blade and pulse until mixed and chopped but not blended. Spread over the apples and dehydrate for 8–12 hours until apples are soft and topping is crisp.

COCONUT MACAROON TART

American	Crust	Metric
2 cups	Dried coconut flakes	180g
1/4 cup	Raw honey or agave nectar	60g
	Sprinkle unrefined salt	

Mix ingredients together in a food processor fitted with an "S" blade. Press into individual tart molds or a spring-form pan. Fill with **Cream Whip** (see p. 132) and garnish with fresh berries or **Sweet Berry Syrup** (see p. 154).

STRAWBERRY-RHUBARB CRISP

American	step 1	Metric
	2 stalks fresh rhubarb, rinsed and chopped	
	2 pints fresh strawberries, washed, hulled, and sliced	
2 cups	Pitted prunes, chopped	260g
	Juice of 1 lemon	
1/2 cup	Raw honey or agave nectar with stevia, to taste	120g
	Sprinkle unrefined salt	

Mix prunes and all but 1 cup of strawberries together in a glass or ceramic dish that fits in your dehydrator. Place chopped rhubarb, 1 cup strawberries, lemon juice, salt, and sweeteners in a food processor or blender and purée. Pour over mixed fruit and stir.

American	step 2	Metric
2 cups	Raw nuts, soaked, rinsed, and drained	280g
1/4–1/2 cup	Raw honey or agave nectar, to taste	60–120g
	Sprinkle unrefined salt	

Process nuts with honey and salt until chopped. Spread mixture over fruit and dehydrate for 6–12 hours.

CHOCOLATE BANANA PIE

Crust

American		Metric
2 cups	Raw almonds or other nuts in any combination, soaked, rinsed and re-dried, or unsoaked	280g
1/2 cup	Raisins or pitted dates, rinsed	70g
1/4 cup	Raw honey or agave nectar	60g
	Sprinkle of unprocessed salt	

Chop nuts in a food processor fitted with an "S" blade. Add fruit, honey, and salt and blend to a sticky dough. Press into a 9–10 inch non-metal pie plate.

Filling

American		Metric
	4 ripe bananas, peeled and sliced	
	4 medium or 3 large, ripe Hass avocados, peeled and seeded	
1/2 cup	Raw carob powder	70g
1/2 cup	Raw cacao beans, peeled and ground to a powder	70g
1/2 cup	Raw honey or agave nectar plus stevia extract powder, to taste	120g
	1 teaspoon vanilla	
	Sprinkle unrefined salt	

Place sliced bananas on crust and press together with clean fingers or back of spoon to make a solid layer. Place remaining ingredients in a food processor fitted with an "S" blade and process until thoroughly blended. Spread filling over bananas. Refrigerate or partially freeze before serving.

BERRY PIE

Crust

American		Metric
2–3 cups	Raw almonds or other nuts in any combination, soaked, rinsed, and re-dried, or unsoaked	280–420g
1 cup	Raisin or pitted dates, rinsed	140g
1/4 cup	Raw honey or agave nectar	60g
	Sprinkle of unrefined salt	

Chop nuts in a food processor fitted with an "S" blade. Add fruit, honey, and salt and blend to a sticky dough. Press into a 9–10 inch non-metal pie plate.

Filling

American		Metric
3 pints	Fresh blueberries, hulled strawberries, raspberries, or blackberries in any combination, washed and well drained	780g
1/2–1 cup	Raw honey or agave nectar with stevia extract powder, to taste	60–120g
1/2 cup	Dried figs, chopped	75g
	1 tablespoon psyllium seed husk powder	
	Sprinkle unrefined salt	

Place all but 1 cup (65g) of the berries in prepared crust. Place 1 cup (65g) berries and remaining ingredients in a blender or food processor and mix until blended. Pour over berries and refrigerate or partially freeze before serving. Serve with **Cream Whip** if desired (see p. 132).

RED SUMMER PIE

Crust

American		Metric
2–3 cups	Raw almonds or other nuts in any combination, soaked, rinsed, and re-dried, or unsoaked	280–420g
1 cup	Raisin or pitted dates, rinsed	140g
1/4 cup	Raw honey or agave nectar	60g
	Sprinkle of unrefined salt	

Chop nuts in a food processor fitted with an "S" blade. Add fruit, honey, and salt and blend to a sticky dough. Press into a 9–10 inch non-metal pie plate.

Filling

American		Metric
2 pints	Fresh raspberries, washed	520g
1/2 pint	Fresh red currants, washed	130g
	4 ripe figs, chopped and de-stemmed	
1/4–1/2 cup	Raw honey or agave nectar with stevia extract powder, to taste	60–120g
	Sprinkle unrefined salt	

Purée all ingredients in a food processor or blender. Natural pectin in the red currants will thicken mixture somewhat. Pour into prepared crust. Freeze and serve partially thawed.

TROPICAL LIME PIE

Crust

American		Metric
2 cups	Dried coconut flakes	180g
1/4 cup	Raw honey or agave nectar	60g
	Sprinkle unrefined salt	

Mix ingredients together in a food processor fitted with an "S" blade. Press dough into a 9–10 inch non-metal pie plate.

Filling

American		Metric
	2 ripe bananas, peeled and sliced	
	4 medium or 3 large ripe Hass avocados, peeled and seeded	
	Juice of 3–4 limes	
1/4 cup	Raw honey or agave nectar with stevia extract powder, to taste	60g
	Sprinkle unrefined salt	

Place banana slices on prepared crust. Place avocados, lime juice, sweeteners, and salt in a food processor fitted with an "S" blade and process until thoroughly blended. Pour over bananas and chill or partially freeze before serving.

RASPBERRY TART

Crust

American		*Metric*
2 cups	Raw walnuts, hazelnuts, or almonds in any combination, soaked and rinsed	280g
1 cup	Raisins or pitted dates, rinsed	140g
	1 tablespoon raw honey or agave nectar	
	1 teaspoon vanilla	
	Sprinkle of unprocessed salt	

Combine all ingredients in a food processor fitted with an "S" blade and pulse until blended. Mold dough into individual serving rounds with a 1/2 inch raised rim on the mesh sheet of a food dehydrator. Dry for about 4 hours.

Filling

American		*Metric*
2 pints	Fresh raspberries, washed and well drained	520g
1/2 cup	Red currants, washed	70g
1/4 cup	Raw honey or agave nectar with stevia extract powder, to taste	60g
	Sprinkle unrefined salt	

Optional: Substitute 1/2 cup (70g) rinsed pine nuts for the currants to thicken

Blend ingredients together in a food processor or blender. Pour into prepared crusts and continue to dry for a few more hours until filling is thick.

CHERRY HEART TART

Crust

American		Metric
2 cups	Raw walnuts, hazelnuts, or almonds in any combination, soaked and rinsed	280g
1 cup	Raisins or pitted dates, rinsed	140g
	1 tablespoon raw honey or agave nectar	
	1 teaspoon vanilla	
	Sprinkle of unprocessed salt	

Combine all ingredients in a food processor fitted with an "S" blade and pulse until blended. Mold dough into individual serving rounds or heart shapes with a 1/2 inch raised rim on the mesh sheet of a food dehydrator. Dry for about 4 hours.

Filling

American		Metric
1 cup	Pine nuts, rinsed	140g
1/2 cup	Raw honey or agave nectar	120g
	Juice of 1 lemon	
	1/2 teaspoon vanilla	
	Sprinkle unrefined salt	
1 pint	Fresh cherries, washed and pitted	260g

Blend pine nuts, honey, lemon juice, vanilla, and salt in a food processor fitted with an "S" blade. Spread into prepared crusts. Top with fresh cherries and serve.

RAW CAKES

Most raw cakes are "patty cakes" made of inspired mixtures of various nuts and fruits, molded into shape by hand or in various bowls or pastry molds. They contain no wheat, eggs, dairy, leavening agents or refined sugar. Beautifully iced and decorated with edible flowers, they are a celebration of life without guilt or regrets.

BANANA-PINEAPPLE UPSIDE-DOWN CAKE

American		Metric
	4 ripe bananas, peeled and sliced	
1 cup	Home-dried pineapple pieces, chopped	120g
3 cups	Raw walnuts, hazelnuts, or almonds in any combination, soaked, rinsed, and re-dried, or unsoaked	420g
1 cup	Raisins or pitted dates, rinsed	140g
1/4 cup	Raw honey or agave nectar with stevia extract powder, to taste	60g
	1 teaspoon cinnamon	
	Sprinkle of unrefined salt	

Cover the bottom of a small mixing bowl with wax paper or plastic wrap. Arrange banana slices alternated decoratively with pineapple pieces over paper lining. Finely chop nuts in a food processor fitted with an "S" blade. Pour into mixing bowl. Process remaining ingredients to a paste and mix with nuts in the processor or mixing bowl. Press half of the dough into the bowl over the banana slices. Cover that with remaining banana slices, and then the rest of the dough, pressing down gently. Cover the top of the bowl with a serving plate and invert. Lift off the bowl and paper lining. Drizzle with **Lemon Poppyseed Icing** (see below).

LEMON POPPYSEED ICING

American		Metric
1 cup	Raw macadamia nuts, rinsed	140g
1/2 cup	Pine nuts, rinsed	70g
	Juice of 2 lemons	
1/4 cup	Raw honey or agave nectar with stevia extract powder, to taste	60g
	1/2 teaspoon vanilla	
	Sprinkle unrefined salt	
	1 tablespoon poppy seeds	

Blend all ingredients except the poppy seeds until smooth. Briefly blend in poppy seeds to mix.

CHOCOLATE ICING

American		Metric
	4 medium or 3 large ripe Hass avocados (Hass work best because they are highest in fat), peeled and seeded	
1/3–1/2 cup	Raw honey or agave nectar (start with less and adjust to taste)	70–120g
1/2 cup	Raw carob powder	70g
1/2 cup	Raw cacao beans, peeled and ground	70g
	1 teaspoon vanilla	
	Sprinkle unrefined salt	

Process the avocado, vanilla, salt, and sweetener in a food processor fitted with an "S" blade until blended. Add powdered carob and ground cacao and process until creamy and chocolaty brown.

RAW CHOCOLATE RASPBERRY GÂTEAU

American		Metric
4 cups	Shelled, fresh, raw nuts, such as walnuts, almonds, pecans, filberts (hazelnuts), in any combination	560g
2 cups	Raisins, figs, pitted dates, or prunes in any combination, rinsed and soaked briefly if hard and dry	280g
1/4 cup	Raw honey or agave nectar with stevia extract powder, to taste	60g
1/2 cup	Raw cacao beans, peeled and ground	70g
1/2 cup	Raw carob powder	70g
	2 teaspoons vanilla	
	1 teaspoon cinnamon	
	1 tablespoon dried orange peel, ground	
	Sprinkle of unrefined salt	
2 pints	Fresh raspberries	520g

Grind the nuts dry to an even powder in a food processor fitted with an "S" blade. Pour into large mixing bowl. Process the dried fruits, optional sweetener, salt, and flavoring with an "S" blade until softened. Add very little water if needed. Mix by hand with the ground nuts, or in the food processor if it is large enough. When dough holds together and tastes delicious, divide in half. Pat first half onto a cake plate (or spring-form pan) and mold into a pleasing shape for the first layer. Spread with **Chocolate Icing** (see above). Cover icing with a layer of raspberries. Pat on top layer of cake. Cover with remaining icing and raspberries.

CHEESECAKE WITH CHOCOLATE CRUST

Crust

American		Metric
2 cups	Walnuts, soaked, rinsed, and re-dried, or unsoaked	280g
1/2 cup	Raw cacao beans, peeled and ground	70g
	1 tablespoon raw honey or agave nectar	
	Sprinkle unrefined salt	

Process walnuts with cacao in a food processor fitted with an "S" blade until it is a crumbly texture. Process in honey and salt. Press into a mold or pie plate.

Filling

American		Metric
2 cups	Raw macadamia nuts, rinsed	280g
1 cup	Pine nuts, rinsed	140g
1 cup	Almond pulp, left over from making almond milk	140g
	Juice of 1–2 oranges	
	Juice of 1 lemon	
1/4 cup	Raw honey or agave nectar with stevia extract powder, to taste	60g
	1/2 teaspoon vanilla	
	1/2 teaspoon almond extract	
	salt to taste, if desired	

Blend macadamia and pine nuts with lemon and orange juice, honey, vanilla, almond extract, and salt in a blender until creamy. Transfer to a food processor or bowl and mix in almond pulp. Spread over prepared crust and freeze. Serve with **Sweet Berry Syrup** (see p. 154) if desired.

CARROT CAKE

American		Metric
3 cups	Carrots, chopped	420g
2 cups	Pitted, soft dates	280g
	1 tablespoon fresh ginger, chopped	
	1 teaspoon vanilla	
1 cup	Raisins	140g
2 cups	Walnuts, soaked, rinsed and re-dried, or unsoaked	280g
	1/2 teaspoon cardamon, ground	
	2 teaspoons pumpkin pie spice or cinnamon	
	Sprinkle unprocessed salt	

Grate carrots, dates, ginger, and vanilla together in a food processor fitted with an "S" blade. Pour into a mixing bowl and stir in raisins. Pour walnuts, spices, and salt into the food processor and chop fine. Mix together with carrot mixture. Press into a 9–10 in pie crust or other mold. Ice with **Cream Whip** (see p. 132).

DATE DIVINITY

I first tasted a version of this at a raw potluck and couldn't believe how simple it was—simple and rich.

American		Metric
3–4 cups	Dates, washed, pitted and chopped	420–560g
	1 teaspoon vanilla	
1 cup	Raw walnuts or filberts (hazelnuts), soaked, drained, re-dried and chopped	140g
2 cups	Fresh berries, rinsed	260g

Process dates with vanilla in a food processor fitted with the "S" blade until creamy. Turn into a bowl and stir in nuts. Place in serving dish and top with berries. Chill to firm.

RAW COOKIES

One day my 18-year-old son came in and smelled something good coming from the dehydrator. I told him I was making cookies. "Great!" he said, heading for the trays. "When will they be done?" I stopped him with a big smile, "Tomorrow morning." Anything you make in a dehydrator is slow food. You anticipate it like Christmas, and when it's finally ready, it's like savoring your presents.

TOLL FREE COOKIES

American		Metric
2 cups	Macadamia nuts, rinsed	280g
	Juice of 1 orange	
1/4 cup	Raw honey or agave nectar with stevia extract powder, to taste	60g
	1 teaspoon vanilla	
	1 teaspoon butterscotch flavor	
1/2 cup	Raw cacao beans, broken into bits	70g

Process everything but the cacao beans in a food processor fitted with an "S" blade until smooth. Pulse in the cacao beans. Drop teaspoonfuls of dough on mesh dehydrator trays and dry until chewy. Serve warm.

CHERRY PIE COOKIES

American		Metric
3 cups	Raw almonds, soaked, rinsed, drained, and re-dried	420g
2 cups	Dried, pitted tart cherries	220g
	2 tablespoons raw honey or agave nectar	
	1/2 teaspoon almond extract	

Process ingredients in a food processor fitted with an "S" blade until dough holds together. Roll into small balls and flatten. Ready to eat, or refrigerate until served.

GLAD ORANGE COOKIES

American		Metric
1 cup	Fresh, brown coconut, chopped	140g
2 cups	Raw almonds, soaked, rinsed, and drained	280g
	Juice of 1 orange	
	Peel of orange, sliced	
1/4 cup	Raw honey or agave nectar with stevia extract, to taste	60g
	1 teaspoon vanilla	
	Sprinkle unrefined salt	
1/2 cup	Ground, golden flax seed	70g

Put coconut pieces in a food processor fitted with an "S" blade. Grate until chopped. Add almonds and continue chopping. Add orange juice, peel, honey, vanilla, and salt. Process until well blended. Mix in ground flax. Form desired cookie shapes and place on mesh sheets of a dehydrator to dry until pliable.

JELLY ROLLS

American		Metric
1/2 cup	Flax seed, rinsed	70g
2 cups	Fresh berries or apricots	260g
	1–3 tablespoons raw honey or agave nectar, to taste	
	Sprinkle unrefined salt	
	Raw almond or other nut butter	

Place flax seed in blender and cover with water. Add remaining ingredients and blend thoroughly. Spread on solid dehydrator sheets about inch thick and dry until pliable. Spread with nut butter, roll up, and slice.

BROWNIES

American		Metric
3 cups	Raw almonds or hazelnuts, soaked, rinsed, and drained	420g
2 cups	Raisins	280g
1/2 cup	Raw honey or agave nectar	120g
	1 teaspoon vanilla	
	Sprinkle unrefined salt	
1/2 cup	Raw carob powder	70g
1/2 cup	Raw cacao beans, peeled and ground	70g
1 cup	Raw walnuts, soaked, rinsed, drained, and re-dried, or unsoaked, chopped	140g

Place almonds or hazelnuts in a food processor fitted with an "S" blade until ground. Add raisins, honey, vanilla, and salt and process until smooth. Blend in carob and cacao. Place in bowl and mix in chopped walnuts. Mold into a rectangle shape on a mesh dehydrator sheet and dry until chewy. Cut into small squares.

CHOCOLATE LOVE BITES

American		*Metric*
	1 recipe **Brownies** (see above)	
2 cups	**Graw-nola** (see p. 58)	280g

Make brownies but do not dehydrate. Form into balls and roll in **Graw-nola**.

GINGER TREATS

My raw friend, Rosi Goldsmith, developed the next two recipes. This one doesn't use nuts, and the next one works without honey or agave nectar.

American		*Metric*
2 1/2 cups	Raw, hulled sunflower seeds, soaked overnight, rinsed, and drained	350g
2 cups	Raisins	280g
	2–3 inches ginger, chopped	
	Juice of 1 orange	
	1 apple, chopped	
1/4 cup	Honey	60g
	Unrefined salt to taste	
	Optional: cloves, nutmeg, mace, carob	

Process everything but 1/2 cup (70g) sunflower seeds and chopped apple in a food processor fitted wit the an "S" blade until smooth. Pulse in chopped apple and cup sunflower seeds so they stay chunky. Roll into little balls and coat with carob or dehydrate and cut into squares.

JAM DOTS

American		Metric
2 cups	Almonds or hazelnuts, soaked	280g
1 cup	Golden flax, soaked	140g
	2 teaspoons ground coriander	
	1 teaspoon licorice root powder	
	12 large, pitted dates	
	Stevia extract powder, to taste	
	Unrefined salt to taste	

Process all ingredients in a food processor fitted with an "S" blade until smooth. Take a heaping spoon of dough, make depression in center with a spoon as circular as possible. Put 1 tablespoon or more jam (see recipe below) in center. Dehydrate on mesh sheets.

JAM

American		Metric
1 cup	Dried apricots, chopped	140g
1/2 cup	Raisins	70g
	1/2 apple, chopped	
	Juice of 1 small lemon	

Process until creamy.

BLACK HALVAH

A sensational raw version of the Middle Eastern sweet packed with the nutrition of sesame seeds.

American		Metric
1 cup	Black, unhulled sesame seeds (or substitute brown for a traditional color)	140g
1 cup	Raw almonds	140g
1/4 cup	Raw honey or agave nectar with stevia extract powder, to taste	60g
	1 teaspoon vanilla	
	Sprinkle unrefined salt	

Powder sesame seeds in a dry blender. Add almonds and continue until mixed and ground fine. Transfer to a food processor fitted with an "S" blade, add honey, vanilla, and salt and process until it becomes a sticky mass. Chill and roll into little balls.

LEMON CHEWS

American		Metric
	Juice of 1 lemon	
	Peel of 1 lemon	
1/2 cup	Pine nuts	70g
1/4 cup	Raw honey or agave nectar	60g
	1 teaspoon vanilla	
2 cups	Almond pulp left over from making milk	240g
1/2 cup	Ground, golden flax seed	70g
	Sprinkle unrefined salt	

Process pine nuts with lemon juice, peel, honey and vanilla in a food processor fitted with an "S" blade until well blended. Add almond pulp, ground flax, and salt and mix thoroughly. Spread on mesh dehydrator sheets to dry until pliable, and then cut into small rectangles.

RAW ICED DELIGHTS

MACADAMIA NUT ICE CREAM

Raw nut milks, yogurts, and smoothies are the base for endless combinations of raw ice cream. For the richest ice cream, start with a thick nut cream instead of nut milk by increasing the proportion of nuts to water when preparing the milk. Another trick for divinely rich raw vegan ice cream is revealed in this recipe: blending a whole coconut with its water to use as a base.

American		*Metric*
	1 brown coconut, water and meat separated from the shell	
1 cup	Macadamia nuts, rinsed	140g
1/4 cup	Raw honey or agave nectar with stevia extract powder, to taste	60g
	1 teaspoon vanilla	
	Sprinkle unrefined salt	

Strain any fragments of shell or husk from the coconut water, if necessary, and place in blender with chopped meat. Blend until liquefied. Strain through a nut milk bag and return coconut milk to blender. Add remaining ingredients and blend until nuts are completely blended. Freeze in an ice cream maker or in a shallow plastic container in the freezer, stirring once or twice before it freezes solid. Serve with **Sweet Berry Syrup** (see below).

SWEET BERRY SYRUP

American		Metric
2 cups	Fresh raspberries or blackberries	260g
1/4 cup	Raw honey or agave nectar	60g
	Sprinkle unrefined salt	

Liquefy in food processor or blender.

FROZEN BANANA SOFT SERVE

You'll need a Champion-type juicer for this, but such a dessert makes it well worth owning one.

American		Metric
	4 ripe bananas, peeled and frozen	
2 cups	Frozen blackberries	260g
	Serving bowl pre-chilled in freezer	

With the blank plate in place, put frozen bananas through a Champion juicer into the frozen bowl. Follow with berries. Swirl the contrasting colors together and serve.

RAW SHERBET

1 fruit smoothie, any type

Freeze in an ice cream maker or in a shallow plastic container in the freezer, stirring a couple of times before it solidifies. Serve partially thawed.

LAVENDER BERRY GRANITA

American		Metric
1 quart	Raspberries	520g
1 pint	Blackberries	260g
1/4 cup	Raw honey or agave nectar with stevia, to taste	60g
	1/2 teaspoon vanilla	
	Sprinkle unrefined salt	
	1 drop pure lavender essential oil	

Liquefy in a blender and freeze in a shallow container. Partially thaw and scrape over the surface with a metal spoon to serve.

RAW PUDDINGS

INSTANT PUDDING

American		Metric
2 cups	Almond or other raw nut milk	460g
	1 tablespoon raw honey or agave nectar with stevia extract powder, to taste	
	1/4 teaspoon vanilla	
	1 tablespoon psyllium seed husk powder	
2 cups	Fresh berries, pitted cherries or chopped peaches	260g
	salt to taste, if desired	

Blend almond milk with honey, psyllium, vanilla, and salt if desired. Layer pudding in a serving bowl or parfait glasses with fruit.

CHOCOLATE PUDDING

American		Metric
1/2 cup	Flax seed, rinsed	70g
3 cups	Water	690ml

2 tablespoons raw cacao beans, peeled

2 tablespoons raw carob powder

2–3 tablespoons raw honey or agave nectar
with stevia extract powder, to taste

1 teaspoon vanilla

Sprinkle unrefined salt

Place flax seed in blender with water. Let stand for about hour. Add remaining ingredients and liquefy. Pour into serving bowls and chill.

CHAPTER 10

TRAVELING RAW

Sooner or later most of us will need to eat away from home. Within a few weeks of deciding to become 100% raw, my husband Thomas and I found ourselves in Kansas City at a Radisson Hotel for a weeklong church convention. Everywhere we ventured around town was decorated with life size cows celebrating Kansas City's stockyard past and preferred menu. This was a big test of our fresh raw commitment.

I had prepared somewhat by bringing a lot of trail mix to supplement what I guessed would be fruit for breakfast and salads for lunch and dinner. However, all the salad bars of Kansas City were proudly groaning with pasta salads, hard boiled eggs, canned beets and other cooked pickles, canned kidney and garbanzo beans (chick peas), and bacon bits, leaving only some old iceberg lettuce, carrot sticks, and the occasional radish for our repasts. We also discovered we were three miles from the nearest supermarket and the banquet waiters at our conference didn't know what to do with us.

Hunger sharpened our wits, and at the next banquet we appealed directly to the chef to make us something from whatever vegetables were on hand without cooking them, with a side of lemon slices and olive oil. We were graced with plates of tender asparagus, broccoli, carrots, and olives on a bed of real lettuce that the other diners envied. One other day we played hooky from our meetings and took a bus downtown to the supermarket, returning with melons, avocados, and peaches. We also found an outdoor ethnic market within walking distance where we bought olives, figs, and five pounds of fresh ripe cherries. Kansas City will one day become as famous for its cherry trees as for its cows if all the pits we planted on the walk back to the hotel survive!

What we learned on that first trip, besides that you can be raw in Kansas City, is that a little planning makes traveling raw not only possible but interesting. Here are some tips and recipes to help you on your way.

BUSINESS TRIPS AND CONVENTIONS

Each destination will have its own challenges and opportunities. Some places ask if you have any dietary needs or preferences, but be prepared to patiently educate them to a new idea: "No, thank you, just because this Jello came out of a refrigerator doesn't mean it's raw." A convention may offer useful amenities such as fresh fruit and vegetables on buffet or snack tables and banquet chefs eager to please. But next time I go to Kansas City, I will be packing avocados, lemons, and condiments with my clothes, along with an array of dehydrated crackers and sweets.

I put a lemon in my pocket when I go to the salad bar or dinner banquet and pull it out to use if lemon slices aren't available. (Thomas has found that fresh lemon juice squeezed over salad bar raisins makes a comforting emergency dessert.) An alternative to lemons as a salad dressing is to mix your own extra virgin olive oil and apple cider vinegar with some dried herbs or Nama Shoyu in a tightly capped little bottle and take that with you to dinner. It's also great to take the healthy salt you've been using. I found a little combo salt and pepper shaker with caps in a camping store, that I fill with RealSalt and cayenne or cinnamon.

Whether to come to the table toting an avocado, salad dressing, and salt shaker to amend your dinner salad or not is something you'll have to decide for yourself. At conferences, I usually wait until the second day, when I've assessed the situation and hopefully talked with someone in the kitchen. If nothing else, I've found my peculiarity to be a good ice breaker and an opportunity to make new friends. If this seems too weird for you, eat in the hotel room first and just have water or tea with your companions.

Here's a list of things that don't need refrigeration to consider taking when you're packing to go out of town:

- Avocados in various stages of ripeness
- Lemons
- Small bottle of homemade vinaigrette
- Unrefined salt
- **Too Skinny Trail Mix** (see recipe p. 145)

- Dried nuts
- Dried fruit
- Dried olives
- Nori to roll up with salad and avocado for a quick burrito
- Dulse or other sea vegetables to crumble over salads
- **Crunchies** (see p. 77)
- Home-dried crackers
- Home-dried cookies
- Raw nut butters
- **Goji Bars** (see below)

Goji Bars

Use gojis for their superior nutrition and interesting flavor. If you can't find any, you can substitute more raisins or dried cranberries, cherries, or blueberries if necessary. Fresh coconut flakes are more work but cheaper than the low temperature or freeze-dried coconut available in some health food stores and from online raw suppliers. Unfortunately, most commercially available "raw" coconut flakes have been overheated in the drying process.

American		*Metric*
	1 brown shelled coconut, cracked, meat removed and chopped, *or*	
2 cups	Fresh dried coconut	280g
2 cups	Raw almonds, walnuts or hazelnuts, soaked a few hours to overnight, rinsed and drained	280g
	2 apples or pears, chopped	
1/2 cup	Raw honey or agave nectar	125g
	1 tablespoon unrefined coconut oil	
1 cup	Raisins, figs, or pitted dates	150g
	1 teaspoon vanilla	
1 cup	Dried goji berries, rinsed	150g

Unrefined salt to taste
Optional: Cinnamon or other sweet spices
and additional small, dried fruit

Chop coconut pieces and nuts separately in a food processor fitted with an "S" blade and mix together in a large bowl. Next, process the apples, honey, coconut oil, vanilla, salt, and raisins to a slurry. Pulse in goji berries but do not blend them. Mix with nuts in a bowl or food processor if large enough, and spread out on mesh dehydrator sheets 1/2 inch thick to dry. When pliable, cut into bars. Store in a covered container or wrap individually for travel.

TAKING OVER THE KITCHEN
WHEN YOU GET THERE

If you are visiting friends or family where you will have access to a kitchen, find out whether there is a blender or food processor available. If so, pack a nut milk bag and some raw almonds so you can make smoothies. If not, you may have room to pack your own smaller "travel blender." You'll also need bananas and some other fruit, so find out what is available at your destination before you pack. Thomas travels with some of our kefir culture in a jar because he likes that so much. You can take along some packets of dry kefir culture from Lifeway Foods instead, which is not as messy.

I'm not kidding about taking over the kitchen. When we visit our parents, they generously pay for whatever ingredients we need to provide raw gourmet food for all who wish, and in turn we do the food preparation. Thomas' folks even bought a brand new food processor to prepare for our visit.

In situations like this where I might have the opportunity to feed others and showcase what a fun way of eating this is, I always bring along my favorite gourmet raw recipe books for ideas. Beginning with one of the raw cakes or pies is a winning strategy that can triumphantly put to rest the oft-repeated question, "But where do you get your protein?"

If you're preparing food in someone's home, save time and expense by bringing with you the things that they don't have, aren't likely to need, or would be more expensive or hard to find where they live. A box of organic dates or high quality seasonal produce can be a very thoughtful hostess gift as well as a source of food for you. Here's a reminder list to help you pack:

- Blender
- This recipe book
- Raw macadamias, almonds, and other nuts and seeds
- Nut milk bag
- **Graw-nola** for yourself and as a gift (see p. 58)
- Unrefined salt
- Stevia extract powder
- Raw carob powder and/or chocolate (powder chocolate first, because they may not have a grinder)
- **Crunchies** (see p. 77) for salads and snacks
- Crackers to share
- Sweets to share
- Kefir culture

EN ROUTE

If you are traveling by car and have lots of room, you can fill up a cooler with whatever you like that you can prepare beforehand and have a picnic on the way. I usually pack a day's worth of wraps (Copycat Burgers with Fixings are a favorite) in a plastic container, air-tight bags of cut up vegetables, a tub of homemade dip or hummus, a jar of raw nut butter, and a dessert. An undressed salad with a jar of dressing will hold for a couple days in a cooler, as will avocados and most fruit, so eat the wraps and dips first. Remember to bring a knife along to cut the fruit. If you have been zealous in making crackers and cookies, you will be very glad to have them with you in some quantity.

Good snacks for the car, bus, train and perhaps plane are tangerines, oranges, grapes, cherries, **Crunchies** (see p. 77), and your own homemade **Too Skinny Trail Mix** (see below).

Too Skinny Trail Mix

Enjoy this as much as you want if you're too skinny or hungry in your raw transition period. I heartily encourage you to dry your own pineapples and bananas. These will be far superior to anything you can buy. This recipe makes a lot but it keeps well. Be sure to drink extra water to compensate for all the dried fruit, and chew contemplatively.

American		Metric
	1 fresh pineapple & 2 very ripe bananas	
1 cup	Dried raisins	150g
1 cup	Unsweetened, dried cherries	150g
1 cup	Dried apricots	150g
1 cup	Dried figs	150g
1 cup	Raw almonds	140g
1 cup	Raw walnuts	140g
1 cup	Raw hulled sunflower seeds	140g
1 cup	Raw, hulled pumpkin seeds	140g

Peel, core and slice pineapple into 1/2 inch thick pieces. Peel bananas and slice into rounds. Dry on mesh sheets in a food dehydrator until mostly dry but still chewy. Mix with remaining ingredients and store in a covered container.

AIRPLANES AND AIRPORTS

With increased weight limitations and security, packing food and supplies takes some forethought. If you are taking any gourmet equipment, put it with your checked baggage. I once tried to bring the business end of a Champion juicer home from my parents' through Chicago in a gym bag and had the bomb squad in a tizzy. If I need a knife to prepare food on my trip, I bring a wooden one from a Chinese grocery store which passes inspection through the X-ray machine.

When I buy my ticket, if meals are being served, I say I am a vegetarian and hope for a salad and fruit. Then I offer to trade my brownie for my seatmate's banana or salad. When the flight attendant comes down the aisle with the beverage cart, I always ask for two cups of water and lemon slices. Presto! Fresh squeezed lemonade.

On the subject of drinks, I also keep some packets of my favorite herbal comfort teas with me because the airline is unlikely to have them. At the airport coffee bar you can usually get a cup of hot water for a small donation to the tip jar. Use it to make your own tea or reconstituted **Soup To Go** (see p. 85).

Two other tips for a healthy and happy raw journey by plane: I've learned that everything goes better if I am thoroughly hydrated before the trip and drink much more water than usual on the way. My other tip is to look for a juice bar while you're waiting in the airport. A shot of wheatgrass in carrot juice or straight up chased with some fresh orange juice (which changes the taste to banana, I swear) is positively reviving. I've found the juice bars in the airports I journey through most. They're not always in my concourse, so knowing where to go saves time.

I am blessed to have the support of my raw friend Rosi with me when I take a long journey. Before I leave for an airport, she gives me one more thing to tuck into my carry on bag—a splendid going away salad. Rosi always assures me that the vegetables have personally volunteered to be a part of my meal. Airplane journeys are physically stressful, so when I sit down in the food court before or between flights (her salads are too dripping with fragrant dressing to open in crowded coach class) I feel especially grateful for the thoughtfulness and love I can truly taste. I've grown to look forward to these meals and appreciate that at least on the first day of my journey, I can continue to eat like a raw empress. Pack the salad in a tightly sealed plastic food container or plastic clamshell you've recycled, secured with rubber bands and double bagged. Bring chopsticks or a plastic fork and lots of napkins. Here's her recipe:

Rosi's Going Away Salad

American		*Metric*
	1/4 head red cabbage, shredded	
1 cup	Broccoli tops, chopped	100g
	2–3 leaves of kale, tough ribs removed, chopped small	
	1 carrot, grated	
	1 apple, chopped	
	1 green onion, chopped small	

	1/2 avocado, diced	
1/2 cup	Pumpkin seeds, soaked a few hours to overnight, rinsed and drained	70g
1/2 cup	Raw apple cider vinegar	115ml
1/4 cup	Extra virgin olive oil	60ml
	1 tablespoon honey	
	1 tablespoon dried herbs: thyme, rosemary, tarragon, coriander powder, fennel, or combination	
	Sprinkle of unrefined salt	

LONG STAYS FAR FROM HOME

Last year I traveled to northern Scotland for a month, including two weeks at the Findhorn community. It was early April, so I didn't expect to find much fresh local produce, and I was right. One raw authority I consulted about international travel told me he never worries about it. "You can always find fruit," he said. While that's probably true, I wasn't sure it would satisfy me for a month, so I took two suitcases, one for clothes and one just for food. On the road, I bought raisins to stretch my trail mix and carrots in a market. At Findhorn, I made **Breakfast Fruit Muesli** (see p. 59) from the breakfast buffet. Since lunch included a raw salad bar, I made two salads and put one away for dinner. I was also given permission to do some foraging in several gardens where I found over-wintered kale, broccoli, spinach, miner's lettuce, mustard greens, onions, herbs, and early edible flowers.

I would have suffered from culinary boredom, however, if I hadn't brought that extra food with me. I was also able to introduce my new friends to some different kinds of food, including my fascinating **Elvis Lives** sandwiches (see recipe below).

On the way home, my now empty food suitcase was refilled with books and gifts. Several years of traveling raw had paid off in teaching me what I needed to know for a successful long trip. Here's what was in the extra suitcase:

• Nut milk bag for sprouting (I could have used two)

- Large plastic cup for mixing soup and soaking nuts and seeds
- Wooden knife, fork, and spoon
- 1 pound (500g) mung beans
- 1 pound (500g) mixed clover, radish, and alfalfa seeds
- 2 pounds (1kg) raw, hulled sunflower seeds
- 1 pound (500g) raw, hulled pumpkin seeds
- 4 pounds (2kg) raw, organic almonds
- 1/2 pound (250g) dried bananas
- 1 pound (500g) dried apricots
- 1 pound (500g) dried figs
- **Too Skinny Trail Mix** (see p. 162)
- 1 bottle raw apple cider vinegar mixed with extra virgin olive oil.
- Small jar of raw almond butter
- 1 clamshell of **Daily Bread Crackers** (see p. 86)
- 1 clamshell of **Simple Sweet Bread** (see p. 56)
- 1 way too small bag of **Goji Bars** (see p. 159) and **Living Fudge** (see p. 129)
- Combo salt and cayenne pepper shaker
- Stevia extract powder
- Cinnamon powder

Elvis Lives

Elvis was famous for loving fried peanut butter and banana sandwiches which may have contributed to his premature death. If only someone had shown him how to make these instead! Here's something I've created that almost everybody likes.

Daily Bread Crackers (see p. 86)

Raw almond butter

Home-dried bananas, dried until pliable, not crisp

Spread crackers with almond butter and lay bananas on top. Press two halves together to pack as sandwiches for traveling or eat open-faced.

INTERNATIONAL TRAVEL

Call the appropriate authorities beforehand to learn what you may and may not bring into the countries you are visiting. Fresh produce is probably not going to be OK, so forget avocados and lemons. I've found dried fruit, nuts, and trail mixes to be permissible. Interestingly, pumpkin, sunflower, mung, alfalfa, and other seeds for soaking and sprouting are allowed. Since they are not for planting, they are not considered agricultural imports. Any of your dehydrator treats will pass. Condiments are also acceptable as long as they don't look like drugs. This is a situation where commercially packaged raw food products may be advisable. A company called Juvo sells a raw food powder in packages that can be reconstituted in cold water, and there is a growing number of raw snack bars available. My current favorite is Lärabar. I suggest you research your destinations online and talk to any people you will be visiting before you go to assess the availability of fresh produce, juice bars, health food stores, and raw restaurants. Then you'll have some idea of what and how much to bring with you.

RAW IN THE HOSPITAL

If all goes well, following a raw lifestyle will make hospital visits unlikely or infrequent. If you do need to go into the hospital, there are two main concerns: avoiding shocking an already ill or damaged body with lifeless food, and supplying the vital nutrients to help heal. If you have time to prepare for your stay, purchase some food enzymes to swallow with the cooked food you may be forced to eat. Food enzymes are different from so-called digestive enzymes which are formulated mainly for meat consumption. Read the label and make sure your enzymes include amylase, protease, and lipase. If you don't have food enzymes, eat as little cooked food as possible. Drink a lot of the purest water available. In most cases, going without much food for a few (2–5) days, if sufficiently hydrated, will not be a problem and may even be a benefit.

Be sure that your physician knows how you have been eating, and if your condition permits, ask for an order that the hospital provide you with at least salads and fresh fruit. Then ask your visitors to bring you avocados instead of flowers.

If restricted to a liquid diet, see if your friends can provide fresh juices from the local juice bar or squeeze some for you at home. I would beg for wheatgrass juice if it were me.

CAMPING AND HIKING

For a car camping trip or picnic, pack a gourmet raw cooler with your favorite dishes. I always include an elegant cake even if it has to be packed in a plastic tub. Eat the fresh, prepared dishes the first day or two. Uncut, washed fruits and vegetables will keep longer. Greens which are washed, dried, and packed in plastic or Food Fresh bags, but not cut or torn, also hold well in a cooler. If the ice in the cooler is replenished, most salad dressings will stay fresh for up to a week. Also, include items that don't need refrigeration from the list in the "Business Trips and Convention" section at the beginning of this chapter. Most of these are light enough for backpacking. Don't forget a sharp knife and a flexible, plastic cutting board.

Foraged wild foods can complement your camp menus or sweeten a hike. I've found berries, mushrooms, sumac, nuts, greens for salads, and tea and sea vegetables on various occasions. Once, while hiking uphill to a picnic spot, I collected wild grape leaves that allowed me to turn our pâté into dolmades. Please be certain your harvesting is permissible and you have positively identified what is edible.

FASTING ON THE ROAD

Without planning, it's possible that your trip could become an unintentional or intentional occasion for fasting. This, indeed, is one way to cope and still remain 100% raw. Be aware that living on water alone or water and fruit will push your body into a cleansing or elimination mode after a day or so.

This is actually nature's way of helping animal bodies recover from illness or overeating. Fasting brings on a healing or detoxification "crisis" that can be ridden through beneficially with lots of water and rest.

However, keep in mind that the stress of travel might not be the best time to invoke a healing crisis. If you are staying in one place for a while, that would be less of a problem. See the chapter "Raw Spirituality" for more thoughts on fasting.

CHAPTER 11

GARDENING IN THE RAW

Imagine being able to wander into the yard to harvest your own fruits, flowers, greens, and vegetables. Nothing can beat the flavor, freshness, and nutrition that will reward you.

If you are already a gardener when you come to a raw eating consciousness, rejoice. Everything you do in the garden will enhance and support your new lifestyle. If you have yet to see that you are a gardener, let me introduce you to this healing, grounding, symbiotic part of a raw life.

I am a gardener. I thrive in connection to the soil. Caring for the life that grows in it gives me both purpose and pleasure.

This is, I believe, both literally true for me and universally true. You may live in an apartment building and work in a city far away from the primal green world. Yet we all wear animal bodies that breathe air, drink water, crave sunshine, and survive on the fruits of the earth, however altered and degraded they may be when we finally consume them.

As long as we live on the earth, we inhabit nature. We constantly affect nature; nature responds. In this sense, are we not all gardeners, albeit mostly unconscious ones?

In cultivating a gardening consciousness, along with some simple practices, we humans reclaim a gift that was always ours: harmony with the natural world, including the natural world in the garden of our own bodies.

CULTIVATING A GARDEN CONSCIOUSNESS AND PRACTICE

Co-creation

We are never alone in the garden even if there are no humans or large animals in sight. Nature sings. We are drawn to its landscapes to find peace and healing because something is there for us. We feel it and love it. We know when it is vibrant with life and when it is not. We may look deeper and know more.

When plants are dead or dormant, life continues. Small fellow creatures, visible ones like worms and bugs, less visible ones such as bacteria, fungi and other microorganisms are all busy going about their purposes. Quiet witnesses, they invite us to be busy about ours.

Some of us see, feel, know, and believe a dimension of nature through inner communion, as well. The Findhorn community, through the work of its founders, especially Dorothy MacLean, has pioneered the practice of gardening, not just with the physical forms of nature but the architectural energies behind them. Dorothy first named them angels and then "devas" from the Sanskrit word for "shining ones." As her awareness opened to commune with the angelic or devic kingdom, she learned much valuable information which was put into practice in the now legendary Findhorn garden. Dorothy, now in her 80s, who has graced my living room leading a workshop and has eaten at my raw table, continues to teach worldwide. Many have learned from her to open themselves up to communion and cooperation with garden guidance. Besides Dorothy, two of my teachers in this field have been Machaelle Small Wright of Perelandra Ltd., and Rosi Goldsmith of Deva Communion.

As you go about whatever garden practices you choose, I invite you to open your mind and heart to the possibility of friendship with all the beings of nature, from elemental beings to spiritual beings. As human beings, we have the potential—some would say the necessity—of taking our place in this larger ecology of life.

What to Grow in a Raw Garden

It is the gardener's prerogative to choose what to plant, whether in the soil, a pot by the door, or a sprout farm at the kitchen sink. Begin by thinking about what you're eating now and what would be convenient to have on hand for frequent use. Evaluate what you might already have growing for its raw food potential, including flowers and herbs.

My garden was already in when I went raw that first June. Unfortunately, I had planted popcorn along with lots of potatoes and eggplants, things that figure only minimally in a raw diet or not at all. A few token lettuces were my only greens, not the collards, chard and kale that I grow in abundance now. Back then, I thought one zucchini (courgette) bush was more than enough and wondered what to do with the extra harvest.

To begin my garden, I make a list of all the things I'd like to grow and then consult both garden books and garden devas for their advice. With every passing season, I grow to know the plants better.

Garden Plants

Here's a list of my raw plant friends that grow in this temperate zone and a few thoughts to give you some ideas:

Alfalfa, for sprouting

Buy seeds in bulk or packaged for sprouts. Soak overnight in a jar, drain, and rinse daily until they start to grow. Give them some light to make chlorophyll, and then store in the refrigerator.

Anise Hyssop

Use the purple, licorice-scented flowers to decorate and flavor salads and desserts.

Apple

Harvest some of the edible flowers to glorify spring salads. You'll still have plenty of apples.

Artichoke

Takes a lot of space for what little you can eat, but the purple flowers are quite ornamental and dry well.

Arugula (Rocket)

An easy-to-grow, cool season green in the mustard family that self-sows and provides sweet, white, edible flowers.

Asian pears

Small trees which produce a big harvest with little trouble compared to apples and European pears.

Asparagus

If you are staying in one place for a while, dig an asparagus bed. The crunchy spears that emerge in early spring taste far better than what's in the supermarket.

Basil

I like globe basil for containers, mammoth leaf for wraps, holy basil for its long season and fruity taste, Genovese for traditional pestos, and Thai basil for Thai flavors. Don't forget to use the flowers, too.

Bay tree

I bought a little plant five years ago and now it is a small, glossy tree that provides fragrant leaves all year round. No more half-used containers of old dried leaves in my spice rack.

Bee Balm

Perennial plants of the mint family with beautiful, edible flowers.

Beets

Good for their greens and roots. Golden beets make great spiralizer noodles.

Beans

Scarlet runner beans have sweet, edible flowers. Bush beans work in containers (so do the climbers if you make a teepee). Purple-podded string beans keep their color in raw cuisine and are easier to find when harvesting.

Blackberries

I don't have to plant these in Oregon; I just prune the ones that are all around me so the fruiting canes are right where I want them. Store the extra harvest in air-tight bags in the freezer.

Blueberries

Another worthwhile, long-term investment to have on hand. They're great fresh, frozen, or dried.

Bok Choy

Crisp Asian greens for salads and wraps. In my garden, the slugs like them as much as I do.

Borage

Its star-shaped, blue blossoms are one of the best tasting edible flowers. It self-sows everywhere once you get it started, but is easy to pull up.

Broccoli

In mild winters, this survives to produce some of the first edible flowers of spring.

Buckwheat

Sprout a day or two for raw grain dishes. Plant in potting soil for cute little buckwheat lettuce, a tasty micro-green. Buy raw, unhulled seeds in bulk at health food outlets.

Cabbage

Pretty much the same, in my experience, as what I can buy, but in a cool garden it is on hand for a long time and I can keep it growing while I use individual leaves for wraps.

Calendula

Easy to grow yellow and orange, daisy-like edible flowers that may winter over in a mild year.

Carrots

Keep in the ground over winter. Gardeners can grow varieties unavailable at the store.

Catnip

The flowers and leaves are as calming for humans as they are exciting for cats.

Cauliflower

If your garden grows plants from the brassica family well, be sure to have some of these. They are beautiful to behold, peeking out from a mandala of leaves.

Chamomile

Either an annual or perennial herb with edible flowers that also work dried for a sun tea.

Celery

I was surprised how easy this is to grow. Lasts all season in the garden and rewards you with a big harvest of flavorful seeds.

Chard

Swiss chard and other varieties last from spring through winter in my garden and even re-sprout from half-frozen stumps. Tender leaves make good wraps. Tougher ones may be finely chopped for salads.

Cilantro (Coriander)

A pungent green worth learning to love and use a lot in raw cuisine. Easy to grow. Also called coriander, for its spicy seeds.

Cherries

Plant a small pie-cherry tree, too, for incomparable dried fruit.

Chicory

Very hardy, somewhat bitter greens with big, smooth leaves that make great wraps.

Chives

Easy to grow in pots on the windowsill or in the garden. Be sure to use the purple flowers in salads.

Clover sprouts

Available as tiny sprouting seeds like alfalfa. Mild sprouts like alfalfa.

Corn

I never knew that it tasted as good or better raw on the cob, especially fresh from the garden.

Cranberry

Will grow in containers and as a matting ground cover in acid soil. More of a novelty unless you have the perfect conditions.

Cucumbers

I like to grow Middle Eastern varieties, such as Amira and lemon cucumbers, which are hard to find in markets.

Currants

Low bushes that tolerate some shade, especially black currants. Easy to grow.

Dandelion

Yes, you probably already have them. Harvest the roots for tea and the leaves for greens.

Daylilies

An easy-to-grow perennial with gorgeous, large, edible flowers.

Dill

Annual herb whose greens and seeds are a good seasoning for pâtés and seed cheeses.

Elderberries

The berries are interesting dried and in syrups, and the flowers are also edible.

Endive

Another hardy salad green that should be in your mesclun.

English Daisy

A very early spring flower that blooms wild in lucky lawns, *Bellis perennis* is edible as well as cheerful.

Fava (broad) beans

A broad bean that likes cool weather. It can be planted in the fall or early spring.

Fennel

I keep my perennial fennel under control by harvesting most of the tender sprouts that come off the rootstalk in spring for salads and soups, and all the seeds in the fall. Florence, or bulb fennel, loves raw gourmet treatment.

Figs

Easy to grow if you can supply the light and heat they need. Tender leaves are also edible and make a stylish presentation lining a fruit platter or under a raw cake.

Fuschia

This pretty flower tastes almost as good as it looks. Decorates a raw cake in a way no pastry chef could equal.

Garlic

Plant in the spring or fall for your own crop of bulbs and green garlic. Easy to grow.

Goji

A vining, perennial, Tibetan native berry. We're learning to grow it here for its taste and antioxidant value.

Gooseberries

You'll probably need to sweeten anything you make with these, but they're easy to grow if you like them.

Ginger

We eat the rhizome of this tropical plant, which grows in my summer garden or in a container.

Grapes

I grow the varieties that are hard to find in stores: sweet seedless Canadice and Himrod, and musky Concord. Use the leaves, too.

Hollyhock

The edible blooms of Hollyhock, along with its sister Lavatera, offer their lovely color palette to our palates.

Horseradish

Turn this root loose in your pasture and forget about it until you need some to wake up your veggies or cure a stuffed nose.

Jerusalem artichoke

Do not bemoan how exuberantly they multiply from small pieces of tubers left in the ground. Make **Sunchoke Chips** (see p. 90) instead and bemoan that you do not have enough.

Kefir

Keeping a kefir culture alive and happy is a form of gardening. Thomas tends our kefir refrigerator farm as his gardening practice.

Kaffir lime

A citrus raised more for its lime-fragrant leaves than knobby fruit. Grow in a pot and bring it inside for cold winters.

Kale

I discovered this important staple of a raw diet is actually edible when I began to grow it myself and learned how to prepare it.

Kohlrabi

A sensational centerpiece on a raw table. Looks like an alien being, especially the purple ones. Makes firm slices for dips and is a good keeper.

Kumquat

Another citrus that lives in a pot on my patio and spends all but the coldest days of our Oregon winter outside. Gives an abundant crop of sweet-tart orange morsels with edible peel.

Lavender

Its flowers are a pleasure to the eye, nose and tastebuds. Needs lots of sun and an alkaline soil.

Leeks

Good raw and dried for **Soup to Go** (see p. 85).

Lemon, Meyer

My two-foot dwarf tree has survived fifteen Oregon winters on the deck and bears 30–50 lemons each year.

Lemon balm

Brings the mild lemon note in its leaves to teas and salads. Grows like a weed.

Lemongrass

A tropical grass with an essential Thai flavor that can be started by rooting a stalk that you buy at the store in water. Grows well in containers that can be brought inside during freezing weather.

Lettuce

Now available in a kaleidoscope of varieties to the home gardener. Easy to grow.

Lilac

Its spring perfume emanates from an edible flower that tastes like it smells.

Mâche

Pronounce it "mosh" and you will be correct. Also called corn salad. A mild cold-weather green that grows in pretty rosettes and reseeds readily.

Marigolds

Some varieties of *Tagetes* species are tame enough to qualify as edible flowers, especially Lemon Gem.

Marjoram

Relative of oregano with a more subtle, complex flavor all its own. Unlike oregano, an annual plant here.

Melons

Gardeners have so many more melon options than supermarket shoppers. Worth learning how to grow if you have the space and the sunshine for them.

Mint

Dozens of varieties, easy to grow in pots. I let it ramble and take over its own space because I use so much of it.

Mung beans

A form of soy bean used for sprouting. Edible just a day or two after soaking.

Mushrooms

Many kinds, including the valuable Shiitake can now be grown indoors by purchasing a pre-spawned kit. A great raw learning gift for kids. Serious mycologists will study how to grow their own cultures indoors or out.

Mustard

For fast-growing greens and edible seeds and flowers. Lots of varieties to choose from.

Nasturtium

Edible flowers and leaves in wild or muted colors. Its spicy flavor goes better with savory salads than sweet cakes.

Olives

I have three little trees growing as much for their vibration and friendship as their promised fruit. Leaves make an anti-fungal, anti-viral tea.

Onions

Top set or "walking" onions provide me with perennial scallions (spring onions). I recommend growing sweet onions like Walla Walla or Maui if you want big ones, too.

Oregano

I have a low-growing perennial variety that is a beautiful ground cover under a cherry tree which stays green year round. Another good container herb.

Pansy

Though among the best known edible flowers, they are never trite decorating a raw cake.

Parsley

I like the curly and the Italian varieties both, as well as the seeds for salads, soups and pâtés.

Parsnip

A sweet white root that holds well in a winter garden. Lends itself to slicing and spiralizing for raw pastas. Grated with an "S" blade, some raw chefs manage to pass it off as rice.

Pears

When the fresh berries are gone, I comfort myself with pears taken from cold storage and ripened in the fruit bowl all winter long.

Peas

Snap peas and snow peas are much less work than the shelling kind. You can also eat young pea plants and tendrils or use them as edible decorations.

Peppers

Raw fooders prefer their sweet bell peppers ripened to a yellow, orange, red or purple color rather than the commonly sold green stage. Jalapeños, green or red are a staple of raw gourmet food, along with other chili peppers for the adventurous.

Persimmons

The fruit of the Fuyu variety is edible when it is still crunchy and holds on the tree soft-ripening through November after the leaves fall. Dries well, too.

Pinks

A large genus (*dianthus*) of spicy, edible blooms that includes carnations and Sweet William.

Plums

Generous, reliable trees. Blend what you don't dry and freeze the pulp in ice cube trays. Store the frozen cubes in ziplock bags to dole out for sherbets and smoothies while you're waiting for the next harvest.

Potato

Determined potato-lovers have spared no effort to render the raw potato as alluring as the deep fried, baked, and boiled ones of late memory. So far, I'm not convinced. Perhaps an irresistible raw potato chip can at least be achieved.

One night the Potato Deva spoke to my friend Rosi and told her this secret: pick them in the dark and ask for their permission first. I have tasted her devic chips and they are very, very, good. Here's the recipe:

Raw Devic Potato Chips

Commune with your plants late some summer evening. When one volunteers, let the tubers come to hand as you gently dig. Place your harvest immediately in a light-proof container. In the dimmest light possible, scrub, slice thinly with a mandoline, coat the slices with olive oil, and sprinkle with salt. Now there can be light to spread the sliced potatoes on mesh dehydrator sheets to dry.

Pumpkin

Grow the sweet-fleshed varieties for raw dishes. Save the seeds for drying with a sprinkle of salt. Naked-seeded varieties are just as easy to grow and their seeds stay fresher than the store-bought kind.

Purslane

A vegetable source of Omega fatty acids, far tastier than fish oil. Grows as a weed and also in more succulent garden varieties. Small lemony leaves good in Greek-type salads.

Radicchio

A red chicory that makes a superior wrap. Sweetest when harvested in cooler weather and very hardy.

Radishes

Don't limit yourself to the perfectly serviceable cherry-red ones. Try black radishes and long white icicles or daikons.

Raspberries

It is possible to find varieties that will give your fruit from late spring through late fall. We let ours take over because Thomas adores them as much as I worship tomatoes.

Roses

Great teachers for those of us on a spiritual path. Rose culture can be simple or complex. For simple, grow *rugosas* which offer fat hips for sauces and teas. Petals are edible.

Rhubarb

One plant is more than enough for most raw gardeners. I had one going when I went raw and now give all but a few stalks away each year to cooked neighbors and friends.

Rutabaga (swede)

Not bad in chips or spiralized.

Rosemary

A woody, tender perennial that's good to have nearby for its unique fresh herbal qualities.

Sage

Lots of varieties to choose from, perennial to annual. Edible flowers. Perennial garden sage is one of the main herbs that raw chefs use to simulate meat-dish flavors.

Scented geraniums

Fragrant, pretty plants in many different scents with small edible flowers.

Shallots

Small, mild gourmet members of the onion family. Quite easy to grow.

Shiso

A frilly-mild annual herb for decorative or salad use.

Sorrel

Sour leaves emerge for early spring salads from perennial roots.

Spinach

Very adaptable in raw cuisine for wraps, salads and ethnic dishes. Gardeners can grow the succulent Savoy varieties with crinkly leaves that don't market well.

Stevia

Grow this intensely sweet-leafed herb successfully in pots or your summer garden.

Strawberries

June-bearing and ever-bearing, OK for pots and containers, especially the delectable, tiny Alpine varieties.

Summer squash

Lots of choices here, all good for raw cuisine and as easy as zucchini (courgettes) to grow.

Sunflower seeds

Raw, hulled seeds bought in bulk-form provide one of the staples for raw sprouts and pâtés.

Sunflower greens

Baby plants that you grow crowded together in flats outdoors or inside, snipping them off as needed to use as salads and garnishes.

Tarragon

Chefs usually mean French tarragon, another easy to grow but rather tender perennial.

Thyme

All it asks is sun and a small space or pot to grow. Lots of good thymes are available.

Tomatillos

If you can grow green tomatoes, you can grow these related green sweeties.

Tomatoes

If I ever could be tempted to join a cult, it would be a tomato religion. Even now, I have a little ceremony when the first fruit ripens. Cherry tomatoes are essential for the raw chef and dry well.

Tuberous begonias

Big, bright flowers that grow in the shade and in pots and are surprisingly edible.

Tulips

Stuff them with pâtés and splash their edible petals in salads to uplift your guests.

Turnip

A humble, fast-growing root vegetable whose hot sharp taste grows with age. Edible mustardy greens.

Wasabi

Hard to find fresh in stores but different enough from its horsey-radish relative to warrant growing your own in pots or wet shade. All parts of the plant are edible, which is good because it's rather small.

Watercress

Sadly, there are few places where it grows wild unpolluted enough to be unquestionably safe to harvest, so grow your own.

Weeds

These are the edibles in your yard that you didn't plant or worry over. Such gifts of nature include chickweed, pepper grass, pig weed, purslane, sheep sorrel, malva, and dandelion. Don't forget you can also put them through your juicer.

Wheatgrass

The most common and probably the best form in which raw fooders consume grains, including wheat, rye, barley, kamut, and spelt, is as grasses. Not being equipped with ruminant stomachs like cows, we must put our harvest through special juicers to separate the rich green plant blood from its indigestible cellulose skeleton.

Much information is available supporting that the fresh juice of these grasses is such a concentrated source of nutrients and vitality that we all should be growing and juicing them.

What stops the uninitiated is the acquired taste of wheatgrass juice. Then there is the unknown learning curve of becoming your own wheat-grass farmer and the expense of the juicer.

I waited two years after becoming raw to fully tackle these issues. One setback was that we burned out the motor of our first juicer when we impatiently overstrained it with too much grass in the funnel. Our new Samson is a tougher model, and also juices vegetables. But if I ever see an old metal hand-cranked juicer in a thrift shop, I'll grab it, and so should you.

After you have a juicer, growing wheatgrass is as cheap as the whole grains and potting soil. In the summer, I even use free garden dirt and compost in my trays, which live outside on the deck.

Growing wheatgrass indoors might even be simpler than sprouting. Soak the grains overnight, drain in the morning in a colander, and then rinse and drain once or twice a day for another day or so until they have tails. Then spread them out as close together as you can one layer thick on top of the soil in shallow containers. Water and cover the containers. Next day, uncover and put them in a sunny window. Keep moist and harvest with a scissors as needed when they are about four inches long. They'll keep growing and even give you a second harvest after the first cutting. Recycle the spent mats in your worm-farm or compost. That's it.

Winter squash

Many varieties, exotic and familiar, to choose from which will keep all winter in cool storage ready for your raw feasts. Serve them peeled and sliced on relish trays as well as puréed in soups.

Violets

Johnny jump-ups and sweet violets can grace salads with edible leaves and good tasting flowers.

Yacon

An enormous plant in my garden with huge sweet crunchy tubers beneath it in the fall. Nice on a fruit or vegetable relish tray and a good keeper in the refrigerator. Save the fertile crowns to divide for next year's crop.

Compost

All good gardens begin and end with compost. As a raw fooder, you will be generating large amounts of vegetable and fruit peelings to return to nature. If you have a garden, there will also be leaves, weeds, and spent plants to compost. Find a corner of your garden for this practice and make an open pile, or buy a rat-proof bin if need be. Raw compost piles don't smell bad or attract as many rodents as those with cooked food scraps. Apartment dwellers can sometimes set up closed worm bins.

Any pile will compost within a year, but artfully maintained aerobic piles break down much faster with the heat of decomposition speeding things up. Aim for a hot pile by making it large enough—at least three feet high and wide—keeping the pile moist and turning it often. See this as a contemplative practice instead of a chore. I love wading into my compost piles to stir them, watching the miracle of compost happen as the elementals of earth, air, fire, and water work together alchemically to create black gold for my garden. It is inspiring to participate in the transmutation of trash into treasure as the raw life cycle continues.

CHAPTER 12

RAW SPIRITUALITY

Spiritual aspirants aim high and live towards their ultimate goal. Life becomes a series of steps taken in the direction of what is apprehended as God. Not, in my life, have I always been directly on the path but always oriented to it, lit by it, and able to return. With such an intention, help comes in many surprising forms. And some years ago great help came to me through discovering that the bread for my spiritual journey could be "living food."

I saw that what I choose to eat has a number of spiritual ramifications. Not the least of these ramifications are the ethical ones concerning how my food choices affect my brothers and sisters near and far, including my relations in the nature kingdoms.

In many ways we are what we eat. It doesn't take a quantum physicist to notice that what we eat affects us in more than physical ways. It affects our moods, our ability to think, to love, and to pray. Avoiding what we know is toxic and choosing what we know is healthy makes as much sense for an aspirant as an athlete. The discipline, mindfulness, and intentionality involved in a raw commitment can be Olympian. I believe that eating raw not only supports spiritual practice, it *is* a spiritual practice, one that is available to all seekers.

The ability to attune to and experience a greater reality is a sought-after prize even in our Western, materialistic society. People might seek such experience in nature, art, sexuality, consciousness-altering substances, and/or religious ritual. But seekers invariably find that what's in the way of a deeper connection with higher Beingness is their own selves. We are too distracted, too tired, too confused, too anxious, too restless, too stuck in physical, emotional, and mental malfunction to taste and see and feel spiritual ecstasy. The challenge then becomes not so much to find God or some Higher Power, but to change what it is about ourselves that prevents joyful communion.

It might seem strange for a theologian to write a recipe book. I've wondered about it myself. Yet my calling has always been to integrate practice with teaching. The great religions demand utter perfection to be fully realized—nirvana, Samadhi, shalom, the kingdom of heaven, to cite a few examples. Christianity in particular—my brand of Godliness—sets forth as its prime example a life of unstinting, all-embracing love at any cost. Adherents must ask themselves, "How do I follow that with all my heart, mind, soul, and strength?"

My whole life has been devoted to answering that question, and eating raw has become a significant part of my life. I hope that these reflections on my experience might be useful to health seekers who are also spiritually inclined or ready to take their search for physical vitality to another level.

ENERGY

I begin here because this is where I first saw the connection between a raw lifestyle and spirituality. Most people, even if they cannot see the so-called health aura, have some sense of the energy given off by others and an awareness of their own energy level. During my first visit to the International Raw and Living Foods Festival years ago, I was attracted to the palpable vibrancy of so many of the people I saw. Watching and speaking with them, it was clear to me that something about their diet afforded these people such an exceptional sparkle. A few of the more spiritually-oriented raw fooders that I got to know also revealed an unusual clarity of connection to inner guidance. Later, when I chose to forsake lifeless food, I experienced both of these gifts myself. And you can, too.

HEALING

Healing involves greater flows of energy: physical healing at the level of more physical energy, spiritual healing at the level of heightened spiritual conductivity, and everything else in between, with all the physical, emotional, mental, and spiritual levels interpenetrating in the whole system. To seek healing at any level is to seek to connect with the source of healing, to become whole, at one, united, joined with All. Eating raw is demonstrably healing on a physical level, and releases enormous energy to heal more wholly.

TRANSFORMATION

If you choose to live in the light of aspiration, you are probably aware of a gentle but persistent inner invitation to step up to a higher, greater life consciousness, the "still small voice" of conscience or inner wisdom. Converting to an all-raw lifestyle in our culture amounts to a major transformation or *metanoia*, and it helped me to recognize this as a spiritual milestone for a number of reasons. One, opening to the spiritual aspect of food allowed the new energy to move more widely in my life. Two, it is difficult—some feel impossibly difficult—to turn against the tide of culture, personal habit and known comfort to eat only living food. Therefore, three, availing myself of spiritual help in prayer and the support of fellow aspirants has been a powerful reinforcement for my transformation.

ALL OUR RELATIONS

All food that we consume as a gift of God is also the gift of our brothers and sisters in the nature kingdoms. Life nourishes life. Most raw fooders, including myself, choose not to take the life of our nearest relations, those with faces. Yet the willing sacrifice of the trees and plants who offer their fruits and bodies to nourish us also deserves honor and appreciation. In gratitude and in turn, the ashes of our bodies will feed theirs.

I was surprised and delighted with my growing awareness of the life energy of plants as I began to incorporate them into my diet while they were still alive. My lifelong habit has been to pluck a fruit or vegetable from the tree or ground or produce bin and consume it as though it were mine because I grew it or bought it. Now that seems inconsiderate of the life I intend to eat, so I am learning to lovingly acknowledge its existence and even have the courtesy to ask before taking. The joy that beams back when I remember to do this confirms for me that life is connected through consciousness. Dorothy MacLean, one of the founders of the Findhorn community, teaches that communion with the plant and devic kingdoms of God is a timely part of human spiritual evolution. The plants not only nourish and heal us, they can teach us from their wisdom how to restore and heal the earth. Healing is not complete until all kingdoms are at one.

FASTING

I have already mentioned that eating all raw has granted me an ease of spiritual connection in prayer and meditation that I had previously only experienced while fasting. I have found an emptiness and simplicity in growing, preparing, and eating living food that makes a space for contemplation in my overwrought life. Since connecting to the Source involves getting past interference in restless minds, emotions and bodies, it's easy to see that having more energy to overcome such internal resistance greatly assists spiritual practice.

Beyond that, converting to a raw diet energizes the cleansing processes of the body much as fasting does. Ceasing to bombard it with difficult to digest substances allows the system to let down its guard and release stored toxins in what may be experienced as a very physical purification process. Many raw fooders are inspired to attempt more extreme fasting to accelerate the cleanup. For me, "fasting" from dead food has been a sufficient spiritual practice of physical purification. There are both physical and spiritual dangers in the temptation to overdo cleansing. If you feel called to undertake a fast longer than a few days, please inform yourself on the subject first.

SERVICE

For the last step in a class I took called "12 Steps to Raw Food," with raw teacher, author, and chef Victoria Boutenko, we were asked to imagine what we might do with the extra energy and time that comes to those who make this change. Many wished to invest their additional vitality for the benefit of others. In fact, the promise of more time and energy to overcome "compassion fatigue" is a very good reason for those of us with a social conscience to embrace this lifestyle.

We are all in this together as communal beings and individual wellness cannot be attained, finally, until everyone is well. Spiritual people understand and welcome this truth with its attendant call to service. I believe that raw fooders already serve by taking responsibility for their dietary health and by consuming fewer of the earth's resources. Sharing our good food and what we've learned about it is also a great service. Let us be prepared to do even more. Investing one's time and energy to help heal the world makes for a satisfying, meaningful life as well as a long and healthy one.

FORGIVENESS

I have spoken much of success in turning from an ingrained, cooked lifestyle to a transformed raw one. Successfully overcoming hereditary eating habits and primal cravings for addictive, but unhealthy, comfort foods will cause your self-esteem and self-confidence to blossom. You will be rewarded in many wonderful ways. I applaud your choice and efforts in that direction.

But what if you fail? What if I fail? One of my early raw heroes, a rail-thin, spirit-bright Sufi now looks like a football player and has been jailed as a sex offender. Others I know, both leaders and followers, have not succeeded in staying on a raw path as completely as they wished.

Fortunately, there is no one to forgive but yourself, since eating cooked food is neither a sin nor a crime! Bringing upon oneself the experience of missing the mark of aspiration is a good opportunity to own up to a personal failing, notice the consequences and move on with the next choice. Self-forgiveness and taking responsibility for our choices is a much needed, and much neglected, spiritual practice.

We might thank heaven for the reality check that our body brings us. Physical perfectionism is an idolatry of the body which prevents us from expanding into a wider spiritual reality and also increases our sense of separateness. Our meat bodies are limited. As sane and healthy and life-giving as a raw lifestyle may be, sooner or later the flesh that clothes the purest raw fooder will wear out, sicken, and die.

Can we embrace our imperfect bodies, our illnesses, our failures, and eventually our own physical death? This, too, is a spiritual opportunity that comes to every life, but quite pointedly to a raw aspirant's life.

Tolerance and humility are related virtues that flow from a forgiving heart. With the enthusiasm of converts, we raw fooders passionately believe in what we're doing. We've made a huge commitment against the grain to walk our talk. Yet there are situations where a spiritually-minded raw fooder may choose to make exceptions. My friend Julie told me she was once in line trying to order a salad to go and discovered she only had a check to pay for it, which they did not accept. The woman behind her stepped up and said, "Let me order you a slice of pizza. I can afford it." Julie tried to protest, but the woman insisted. The person behind the counter heard the exchange, returned the stranger's money and said, "That's all right. We throw away extra pizza all the time. Here's a couple slices." Julie didn't mention she really wanted raw food instead and sincerely thanked her benefactors. Those pizza slices became holy food both by gracious giving and gracious receiving. For spiritual folk, it's ultimately not about the enzymes, it's about the love.

GRATITUDE

Since becoming raw, I have become mindful not only to give thanks for the food, but also to the food and even with the food. When the food we take in thrums with life, so do we. Grateful, we may open our hearts, adding love to love. As we embrace the flow of life blessing us, gratitude grows to joy and joy rises to ecstasy. Whatever your path, may you be blessed with vitality. And may you be blessed with Life beyond vitality. Thank you.

BIBLIOGRAPHY

Baird, Lori, *The Complete Book of Raw Food*. Healthy Living Books

Boutenko, Sergei and Valya, *Eating Without Heating*. Raw Family Press

Boutenko, Victoria, *12 Steps to Raw Food*. Raw Family Press

Chavez, Thomas, *Body Electronics: Vital Steps to Physical Regeneration*. North Atlantic Books

Cousens, Gabriel, *Rainbow Green Live-Food Cuisine*. North Atlantic Books

Creasy, Rosalind, *The Edible Flower Garden*. Periplus

Findhorn Community, *The Findhorn Garden*. Findhorn Press

Juliano, *Raw—the Uncook Book*. Regan Books

MacLean, Dorothy, *Choices of Love*. Lindisfarne Books
                    To Hear the Angels Sing. Lindisfarne Books

Rhio, *Hooked on Raw*. Beso Entertainment

Trotter, Charlie and Roxanne Klein, *Raw*. Ten Speed Press

Wright, Machaelle Small,
        Behaving As if the God in all Life Mattered. Perelandra   Ltd.
        Perelandra Garden Workbook I and II. Perelandra Ltd.

Appendix

• *Online sources of raw food information, equipment and supplies:*

www.rawfamily.com

www.rawchef.org

http://users.chariot.net.au/~dna/kefirpage.html (Dom's kefir in-site)

www.gojuvo.com

www.eatraw.com

www.larabar.com

www.livingtreecommunity.com

www.purejoylivingfoods.com

www.rawfood.com

www.rawfoodinfo.com

www.rawgourmet.com

www.sunorganic.com

www.thegardendiet.com

• *For information about gardening in communication with the nature kingdoms:*

www.devacommunion.org

INDEX OF RECIPES